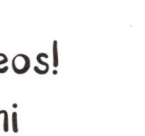

Don't forget to tag us in pictures and videos!
Instagram and Facebook @MirculousOmni
www.miraculousjourneys.org

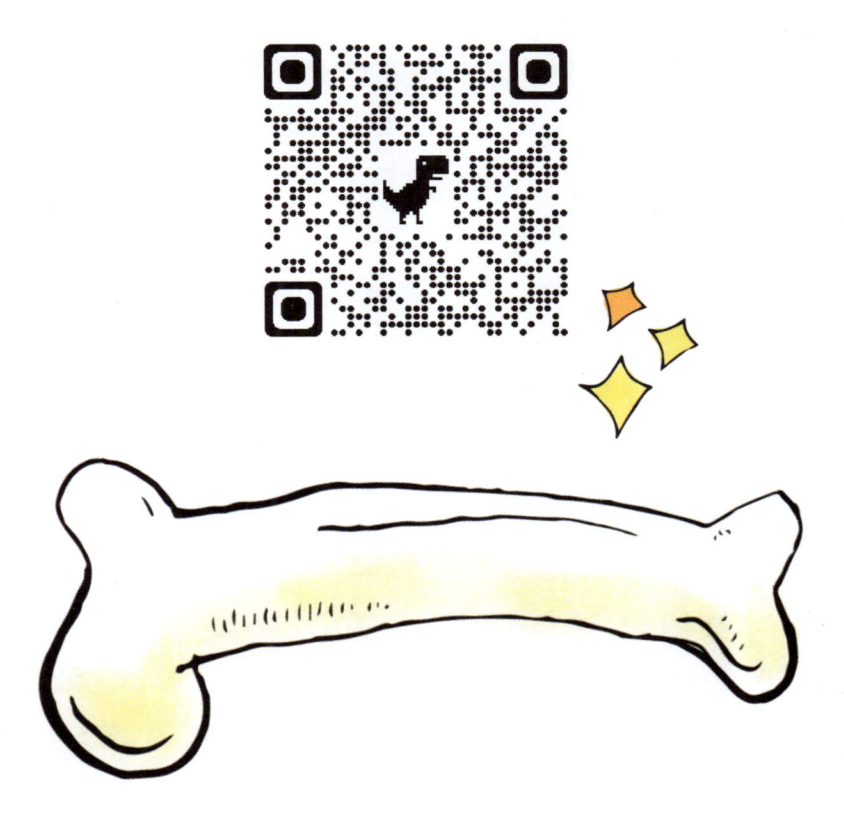

Copyright © 2021 by Dr. Steven Patton

All rights reserved. No part of this book may be reproduced or used in any manner without written permission of the copyright owner except for the use of quotations in a book review.

ISBN 979-8-9850241-0-4

I remember it just like it was yesterday. Fragrances of sweet, melted apple cinnamon wax filled the room as the off-key notes from our miniature electric piano echoed in the background. My daughter and I would create silly songs and poems in my shameless attempt to teach a five-year-old anatomy. I would smile with admiration as she fumbled and stuttered over vocabulary words that most adults could barely pronounce or even understand, but hey, we were having fun!

It was soon that I realized that our rhythmic adventures were paying off; not only was she able to pronounce her anatomy words, but she was able to point out their location! We made an awesome duet but an even stronger bond. This is when I knew I wanted to share our experience with parents and children across the world.

I CAN BE anything. ANYTHING THAT I want.

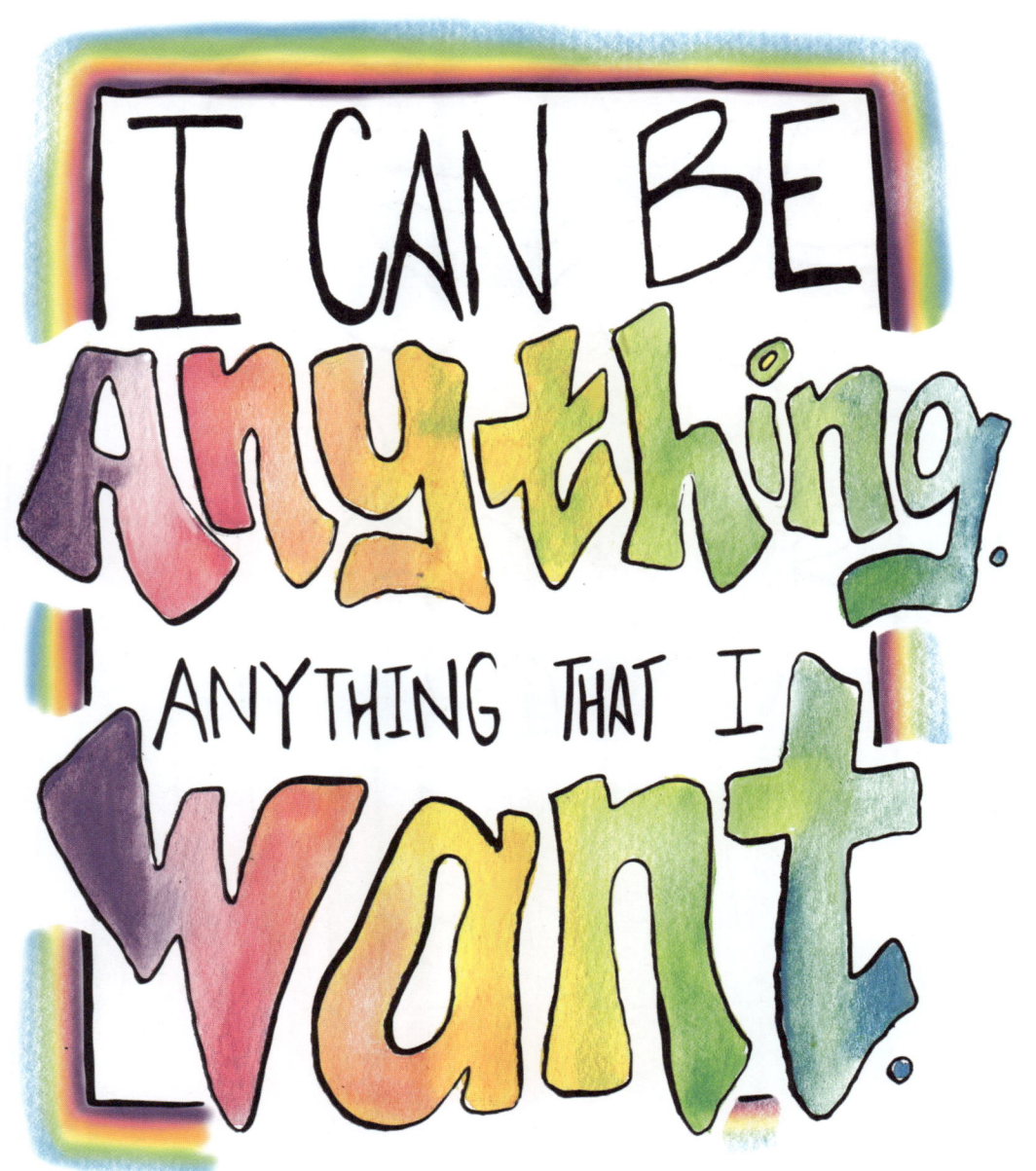

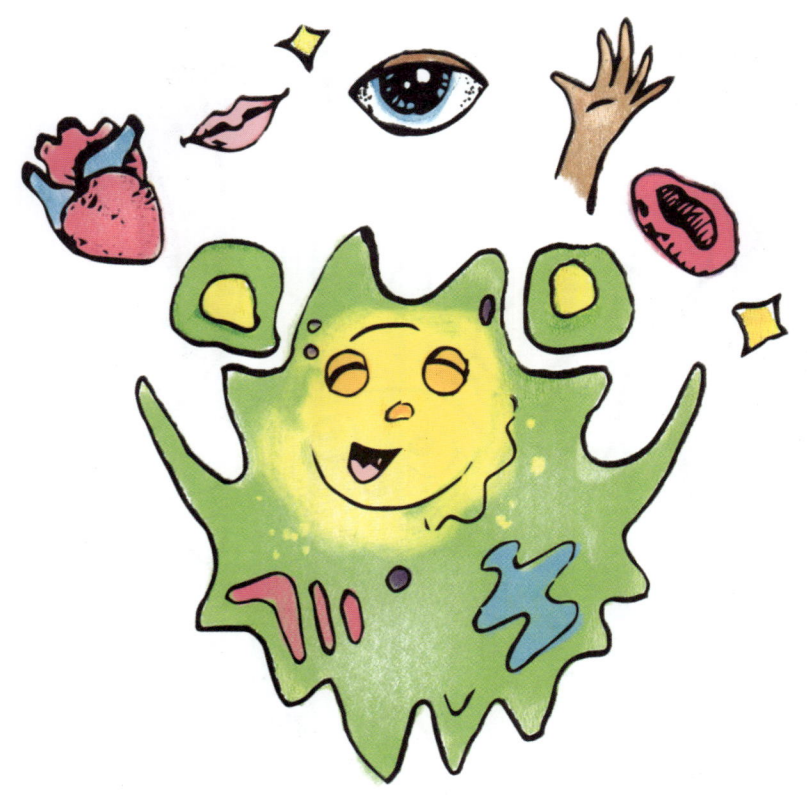

I can have anything by working hard up front!

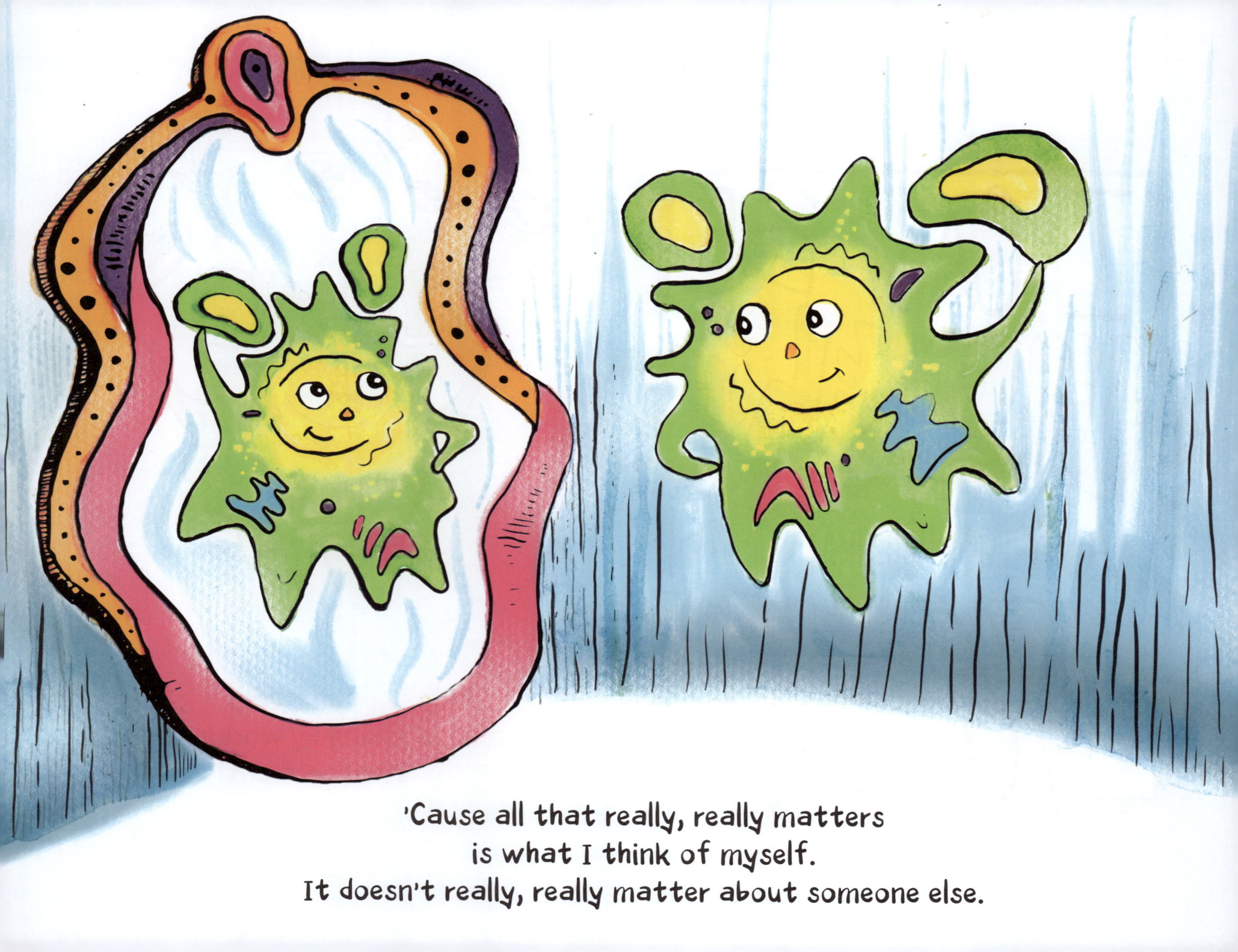

'Cause all that really, really matters
is what I think of myself.
It doesn't really, really matter about someone else.

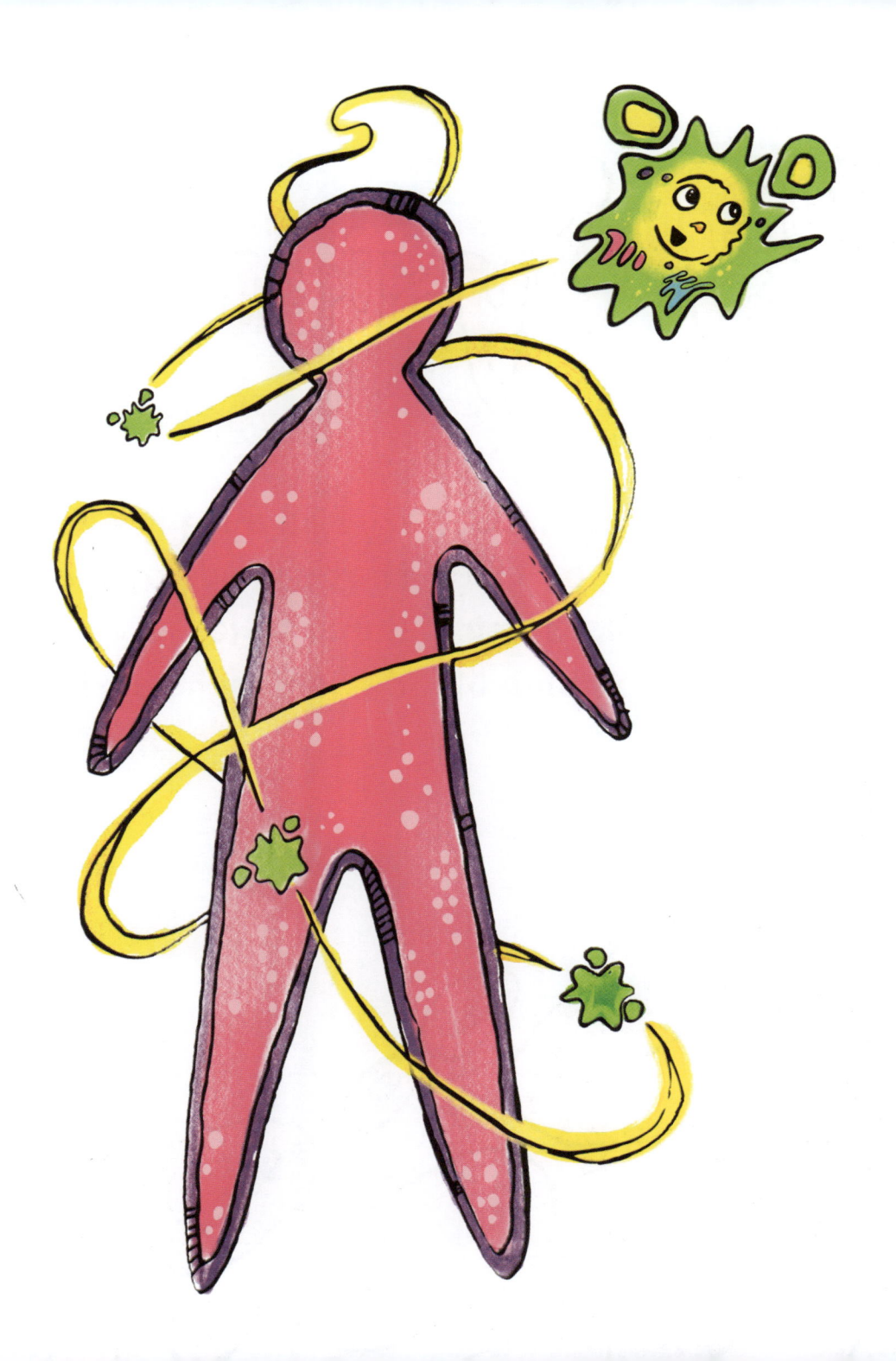

Here's the story of **OMNI**,
An omnipotent (um-ni-puh-tnt) cell,
Who must travel the body
with stories to tell.
It needs your assistance,
so you can decide,
in which part of the body
it needs to reside.
There are different lessons,
that each system brings,
since Omni the cell can
become anything!

Circulatory System
(sur-kyuh-luh-taw-ree)

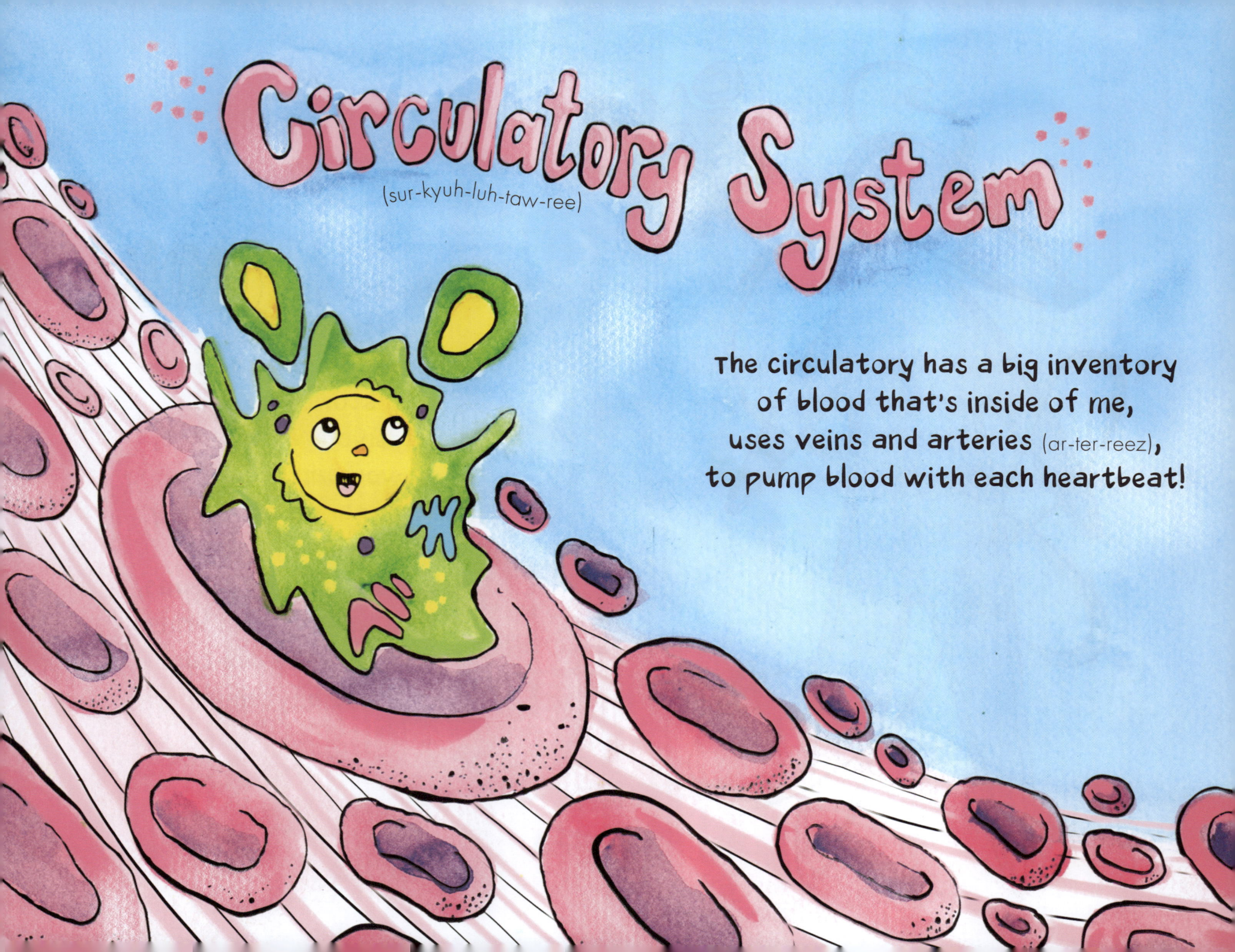

The circulatory has a big inventory of blood that's inside of me, uses veins and arteries (ar-ter-reez), to pump blood with each heartbeat!

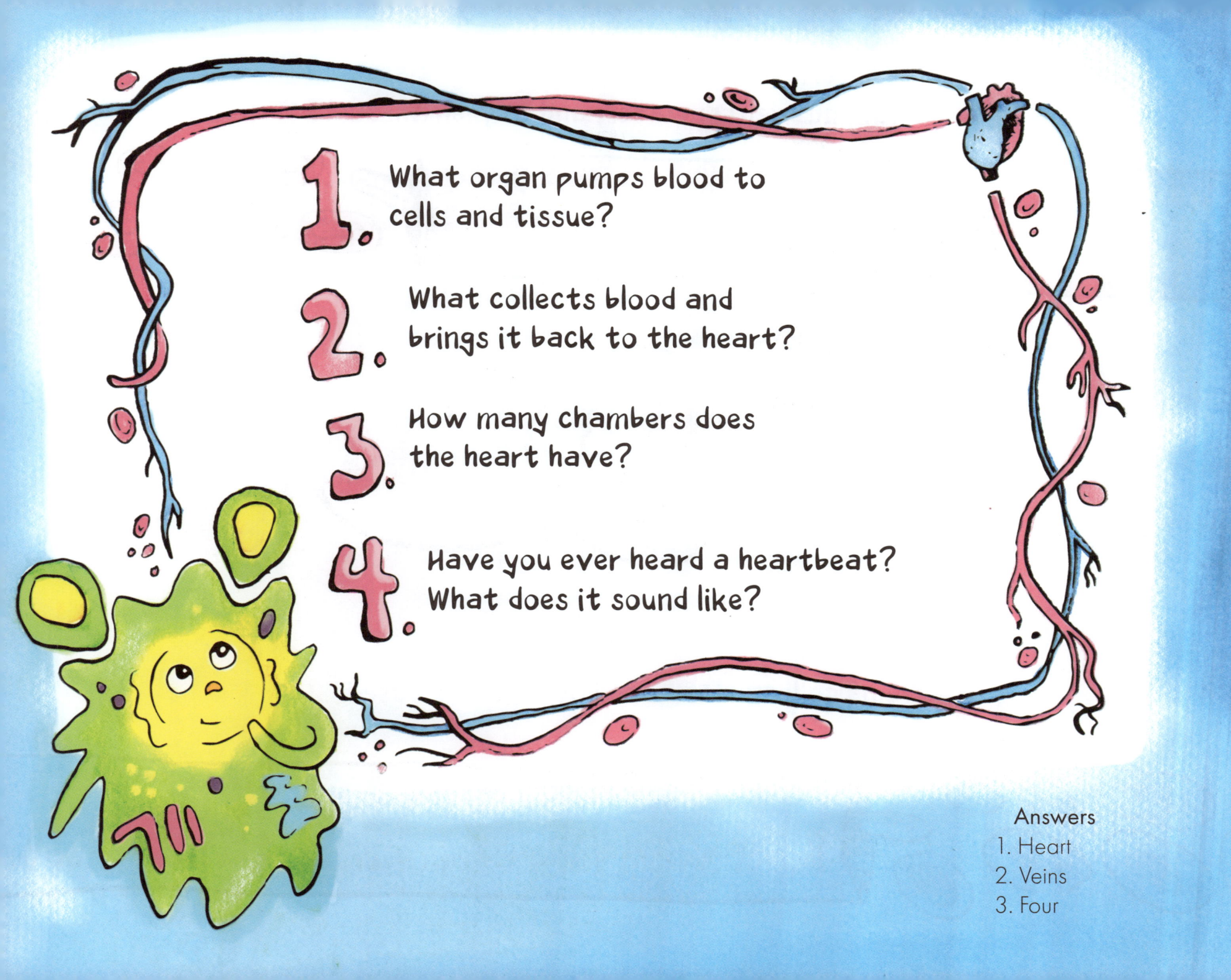

1. What organ pumps blood to cells and tissue?

2. What collects blood and brings it back to the heart?

3. How many chambers does the heart have?

4. Have you ever heard a heartbeat? What does it sound like?

Answers
1. Heart
2. Veins
3. Four

Arteries move blood to cells and tissue,
bring nutrients, water, and oxygen through.

Blood is part plasma, H_2O and O_2.

Veins collect blood once everything's used.

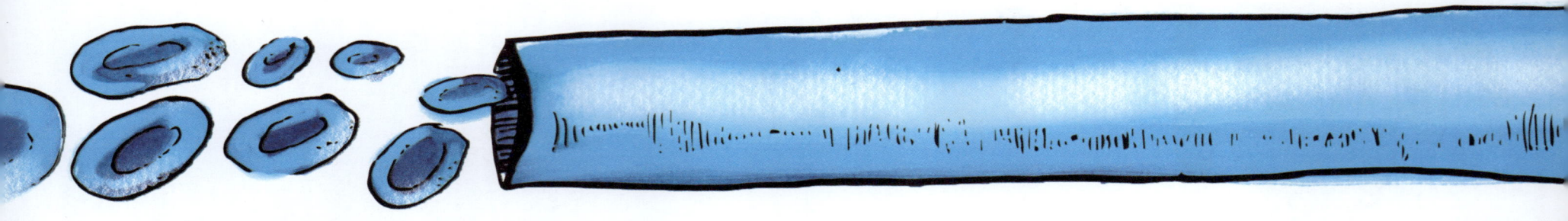

From liver to lungs and the rest of the body, veins collect blood for the heart's favorite hobby. Fills up the four chambers inside of the chest. Blood comes from the right and pumps out through the left.

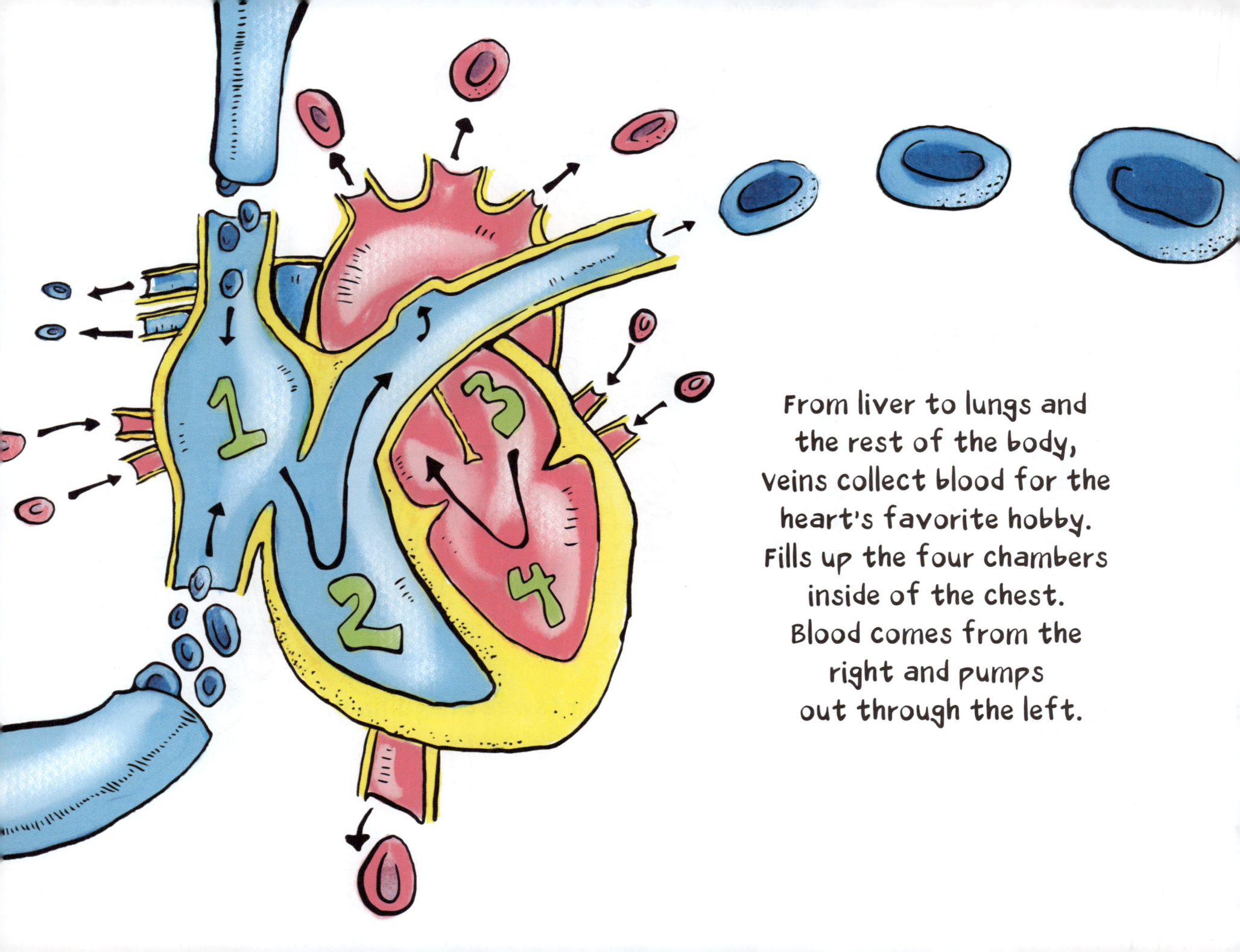

Digestive System

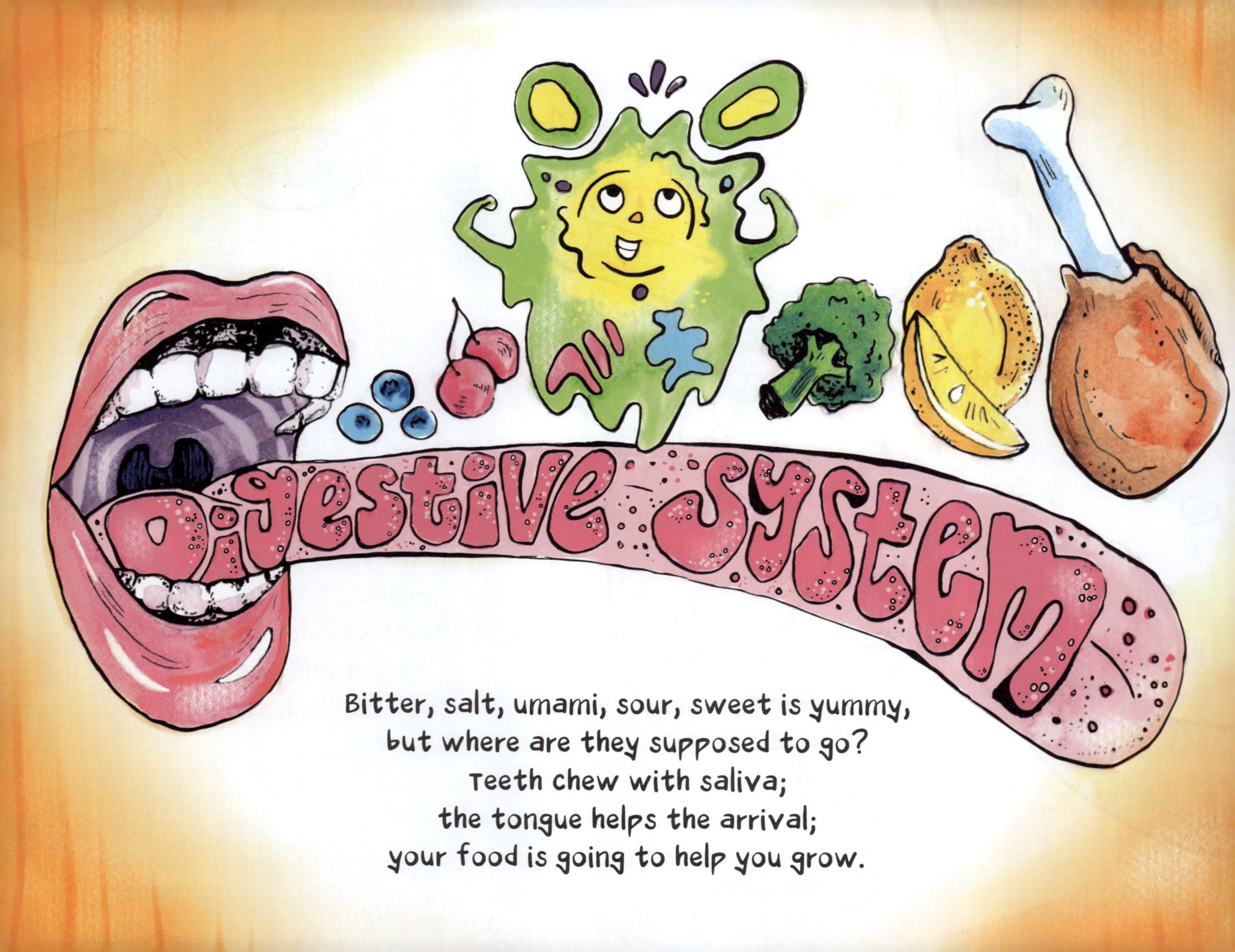

Bitter, salt, umami, sour, sweet is yummy,
but where are they supposed to go?
Teeth chew with saliva;
the tongue helps the arrival;
your food is going to help you grow.

1. What are the five basic tastes?

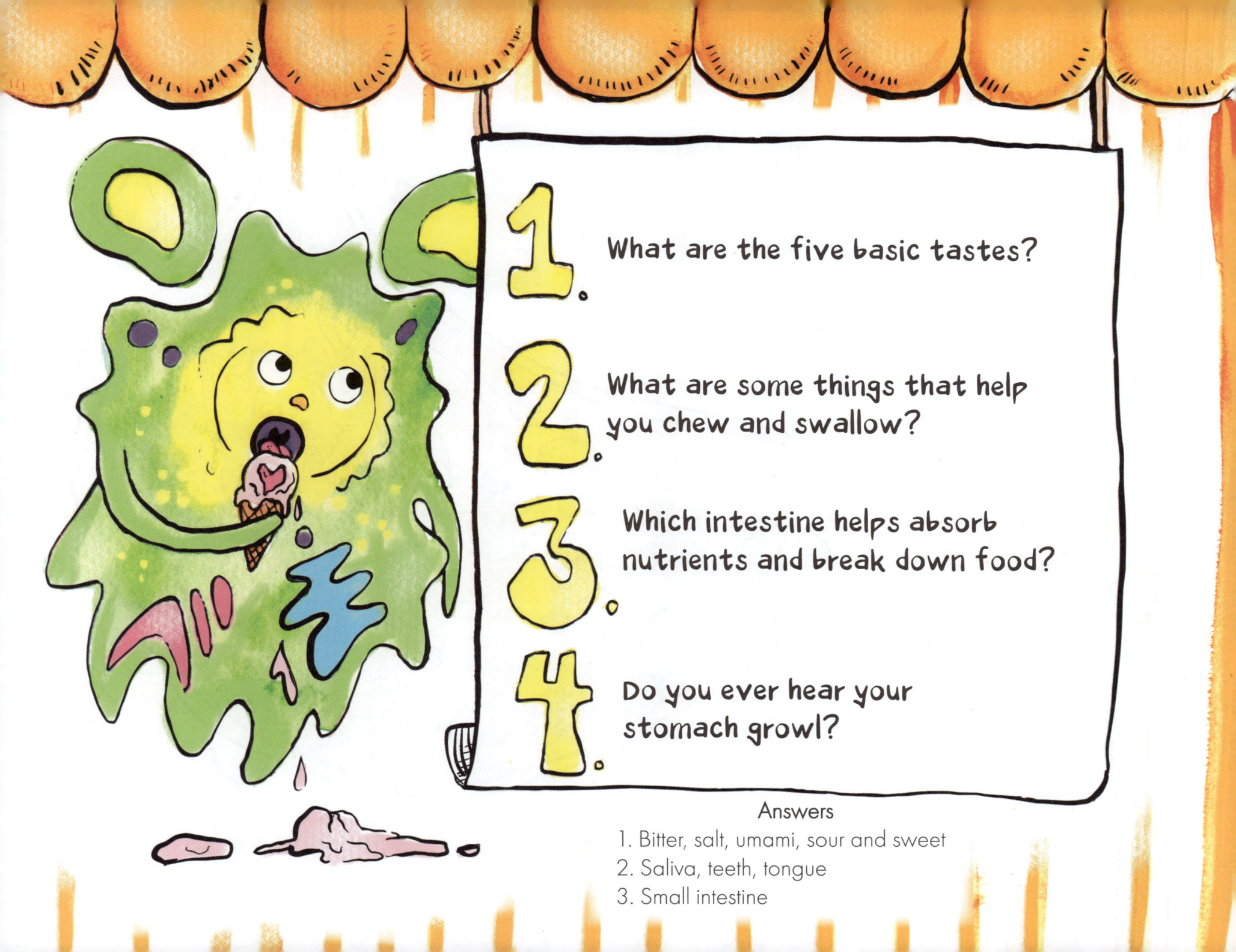

2. What are some things that help you chew and swallow?

3. Which intestine helps absorb nutrients and break down food?

4. Do you ever hear your stomach growl?

Answers
1. Bitter, salt, umami, sour and sweet
2. Saliva, teeth, tongue
3. Small intestine

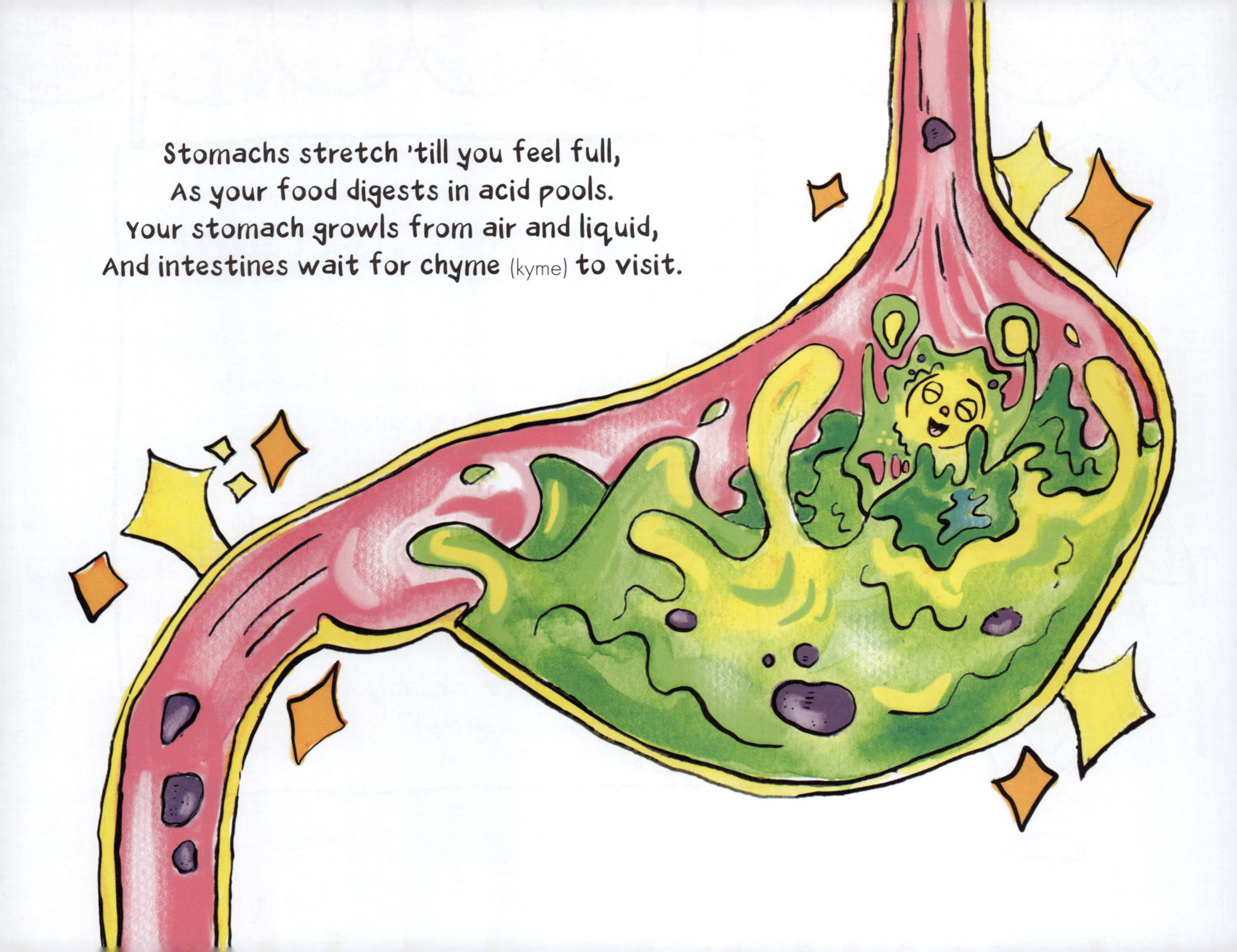

Stomachs stretch 'till you feel full,
As your food digests in acid pools.
Your stomach growls from air and liquid,
And intestines wait for chyme (kyme) to visit.

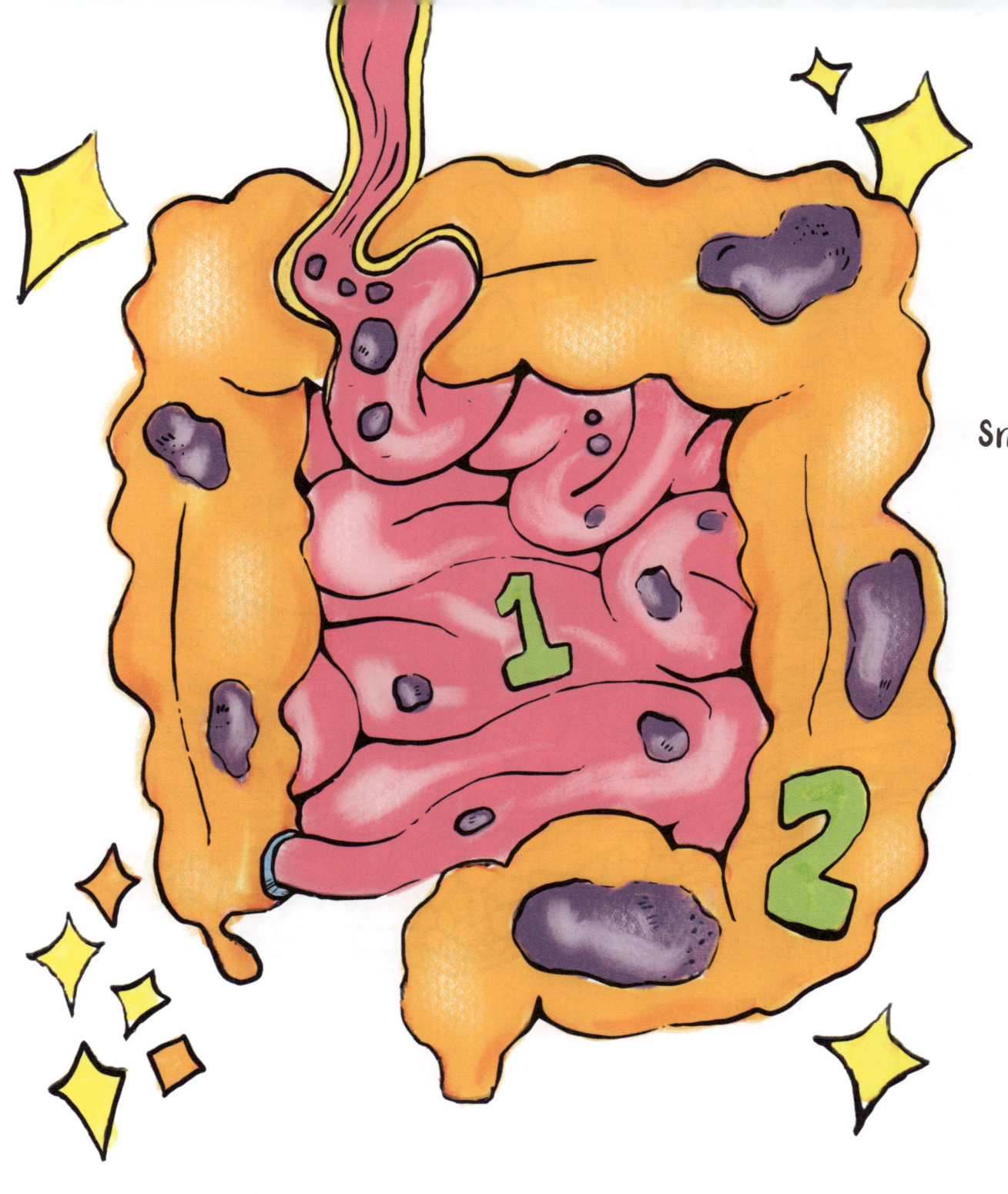

Small intestines, large ones too —
Question is, what does each one do?
Small is one and large is two,
The order of how your food goes through.

Small has enzymes to break down food.
Nutrients are absorbed by you.
The rest is fiber that can't get through,
so the large intestine turns that to poo.

Integumentary System
(In-te-gu-men-tary)

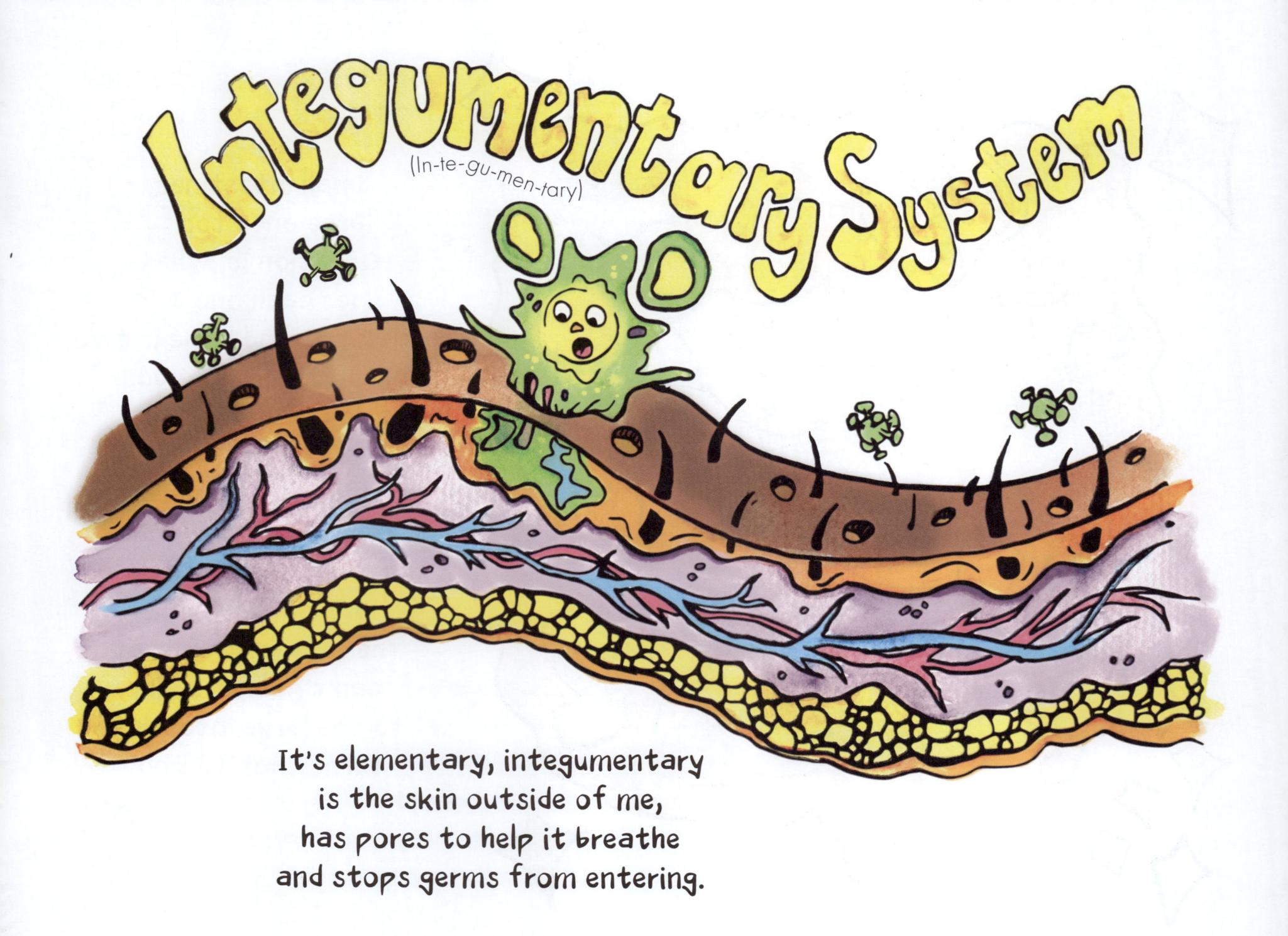

It's elementary, integumentary
is the skin outside of me,
has pores to help it breathe
and stops germs from entering.

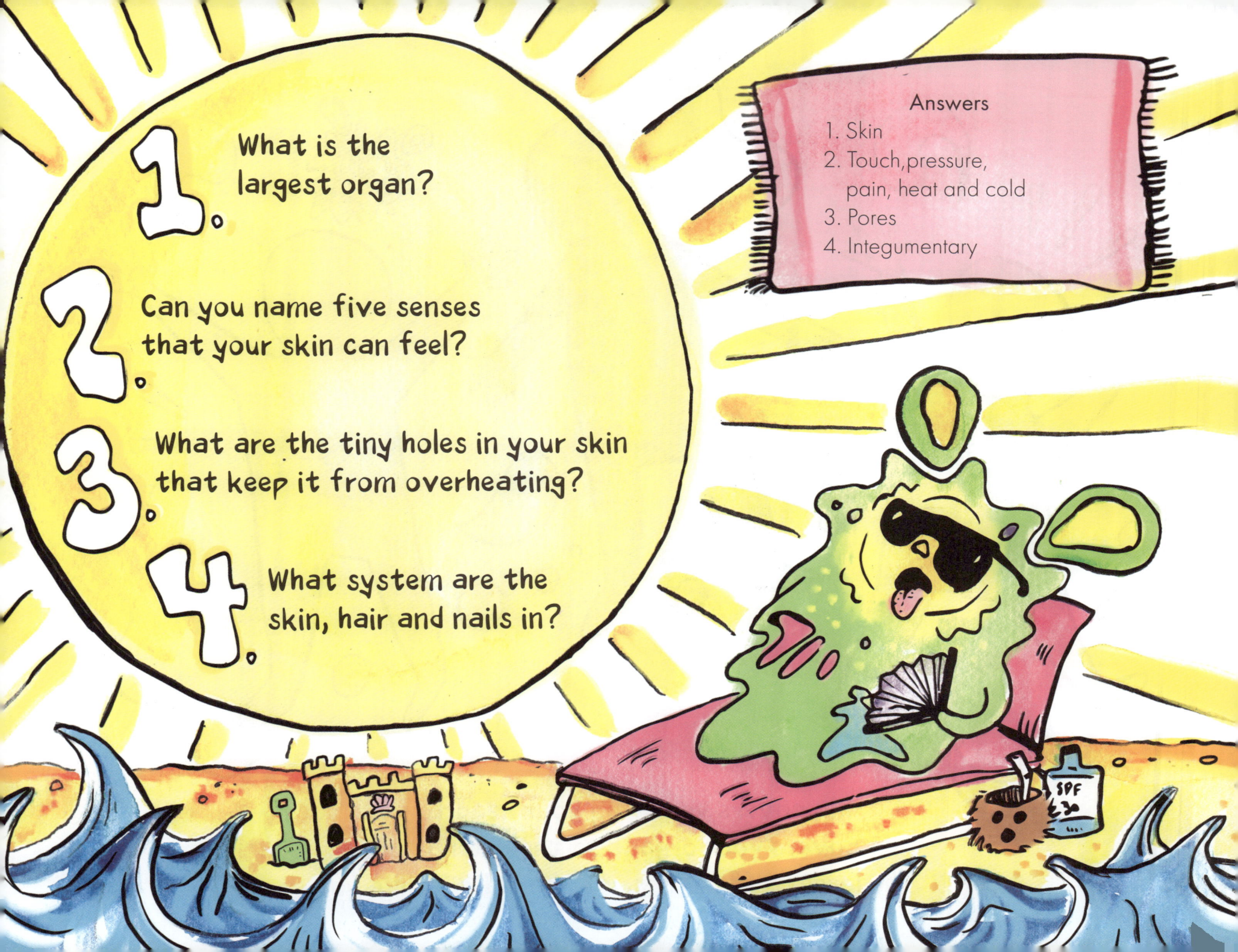

1. What is the largest organ?

2. Can you name five senses that your skin can feel?

3. What are the tiny holes in your skin that keep it from overheating?

4. What system are the skin, hair and nails in?

Answers
1. Skin
2. Touch, pressure, pain, heat and cold
3. Pores
4. Integumentary

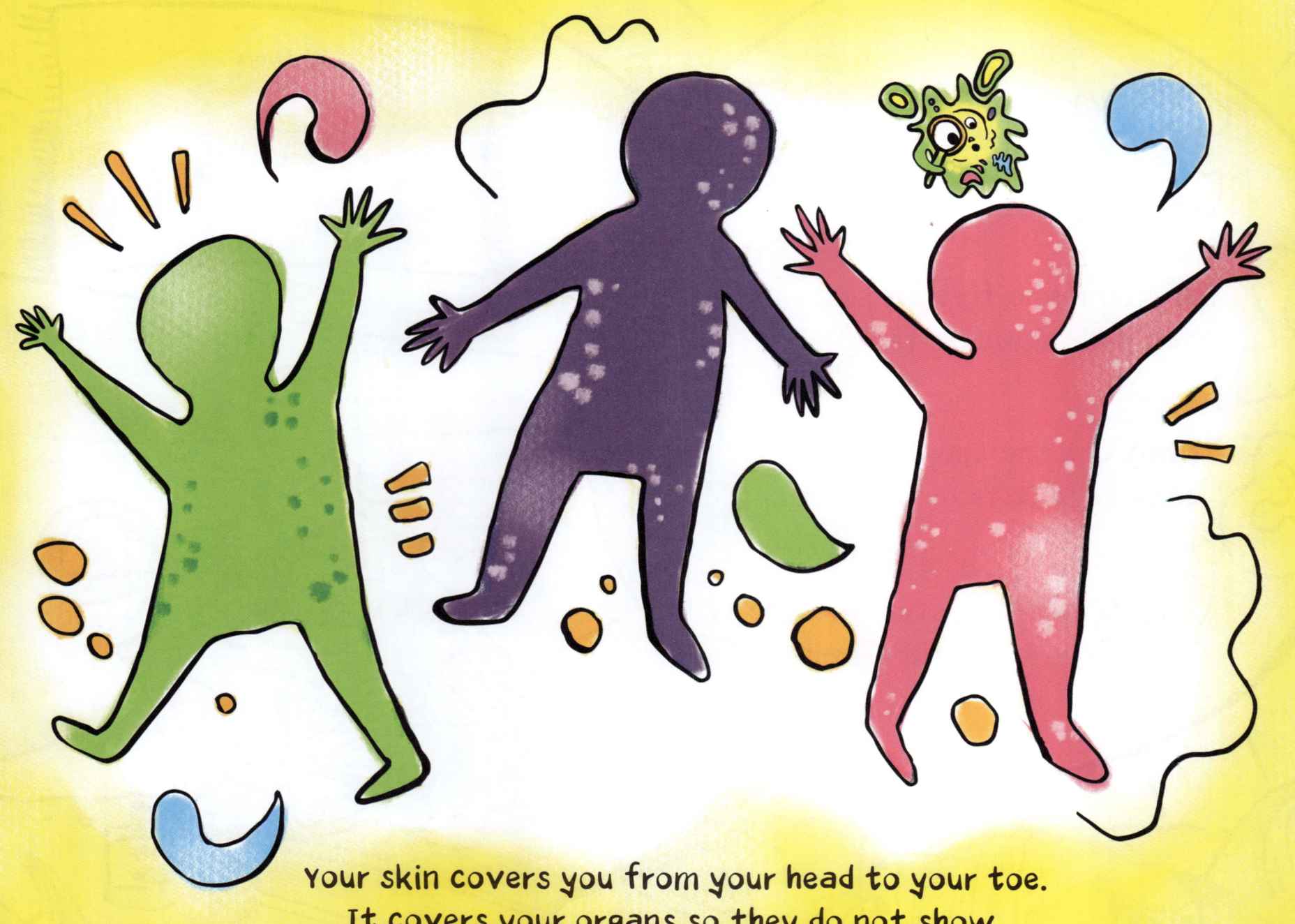

Your skin covers you from your head to your toe.
It covers your organs so they do not show.
The largest of organs, its shaped just like you.

Your hair and your nails are a part of it too.
It likes to use neurons, so you can behold,
touch, pressure, pain, heat and the cold.

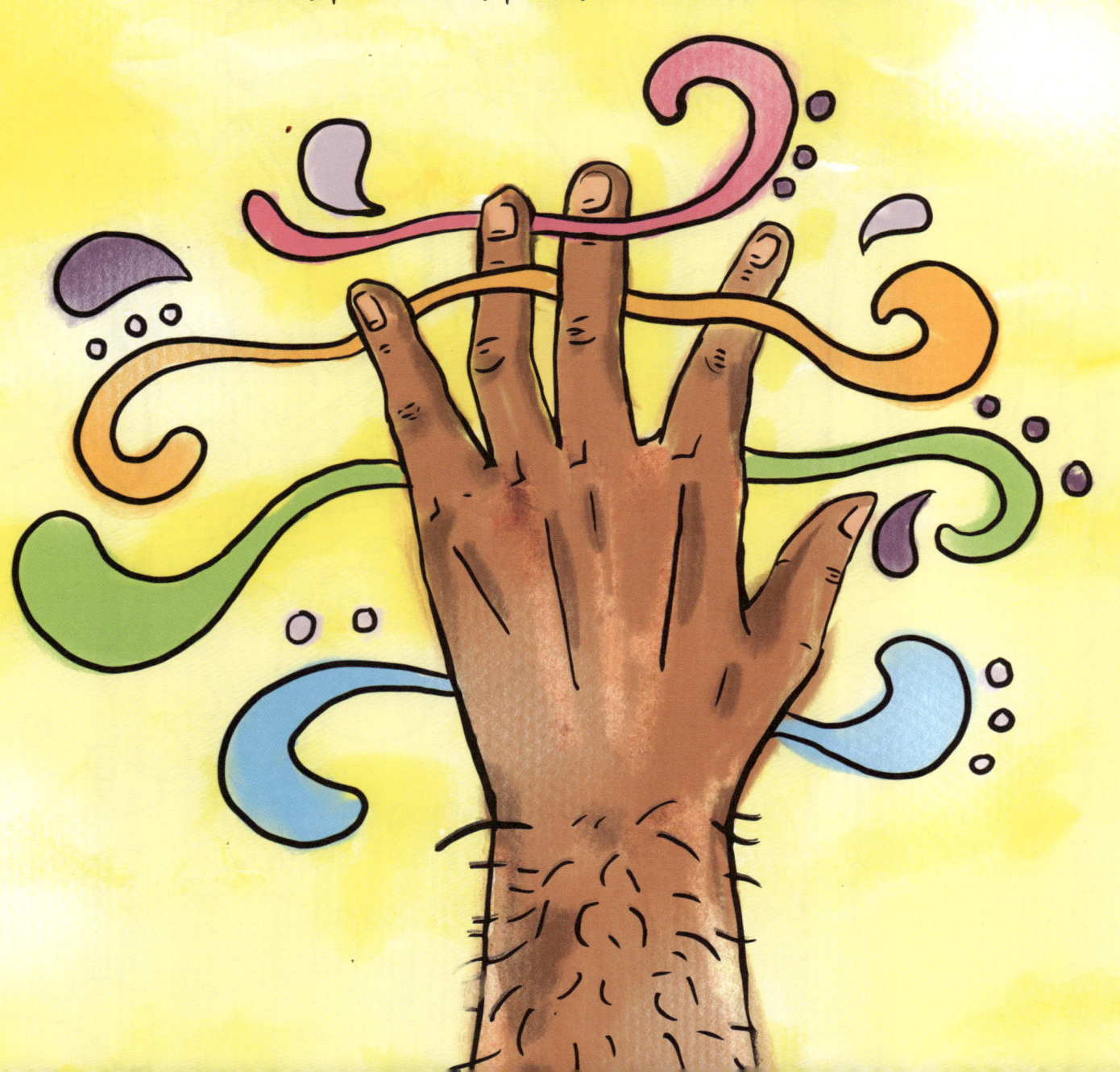

Lymphatic Immune System
(lum-fa-tuhk)

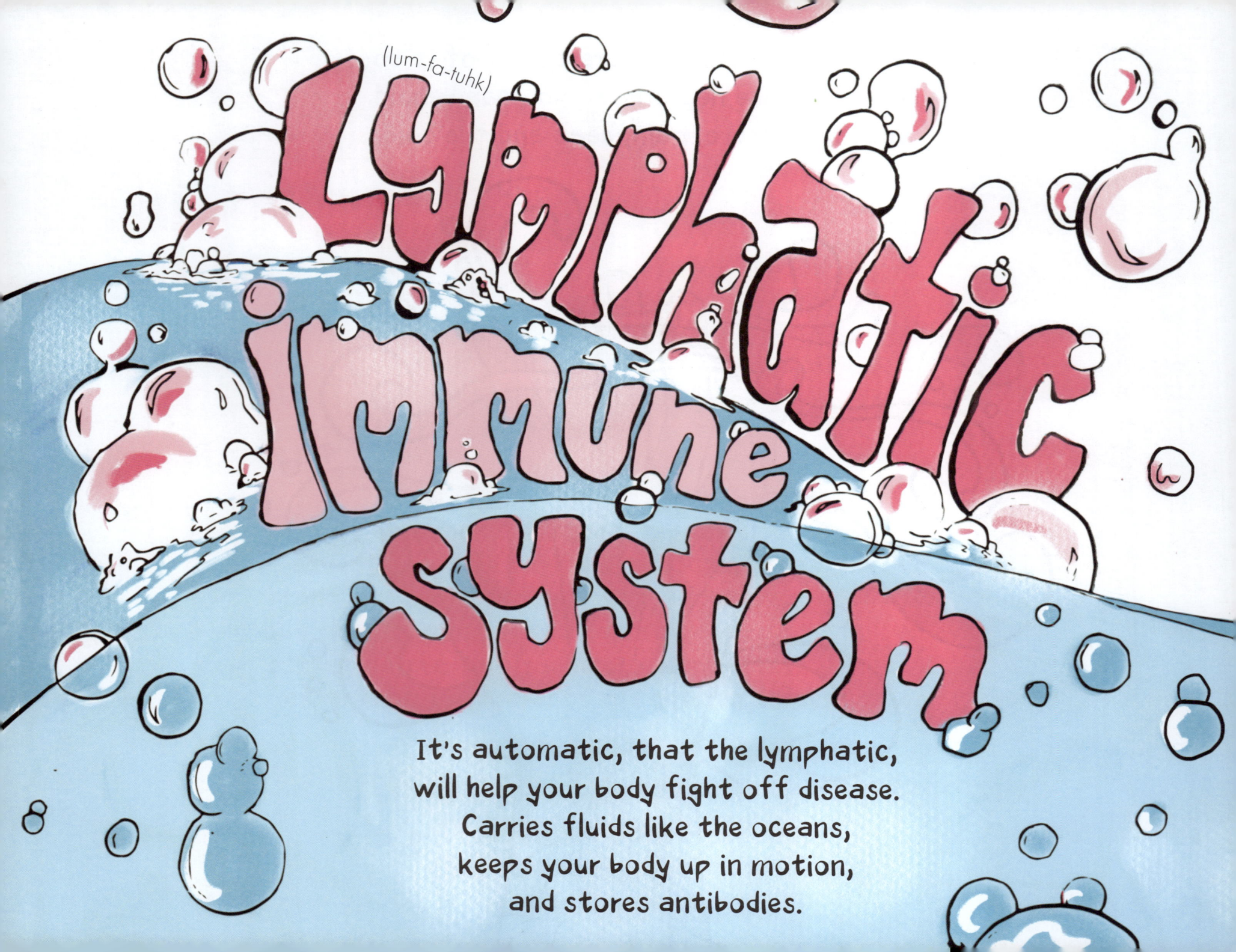

It's automatic, that the lymphatic,
will help your body fight off disease.
Carries fluids like the oceans,
keeps your body up in motion,
and stores antibodies.

1. What system helps fight viruses and germs?

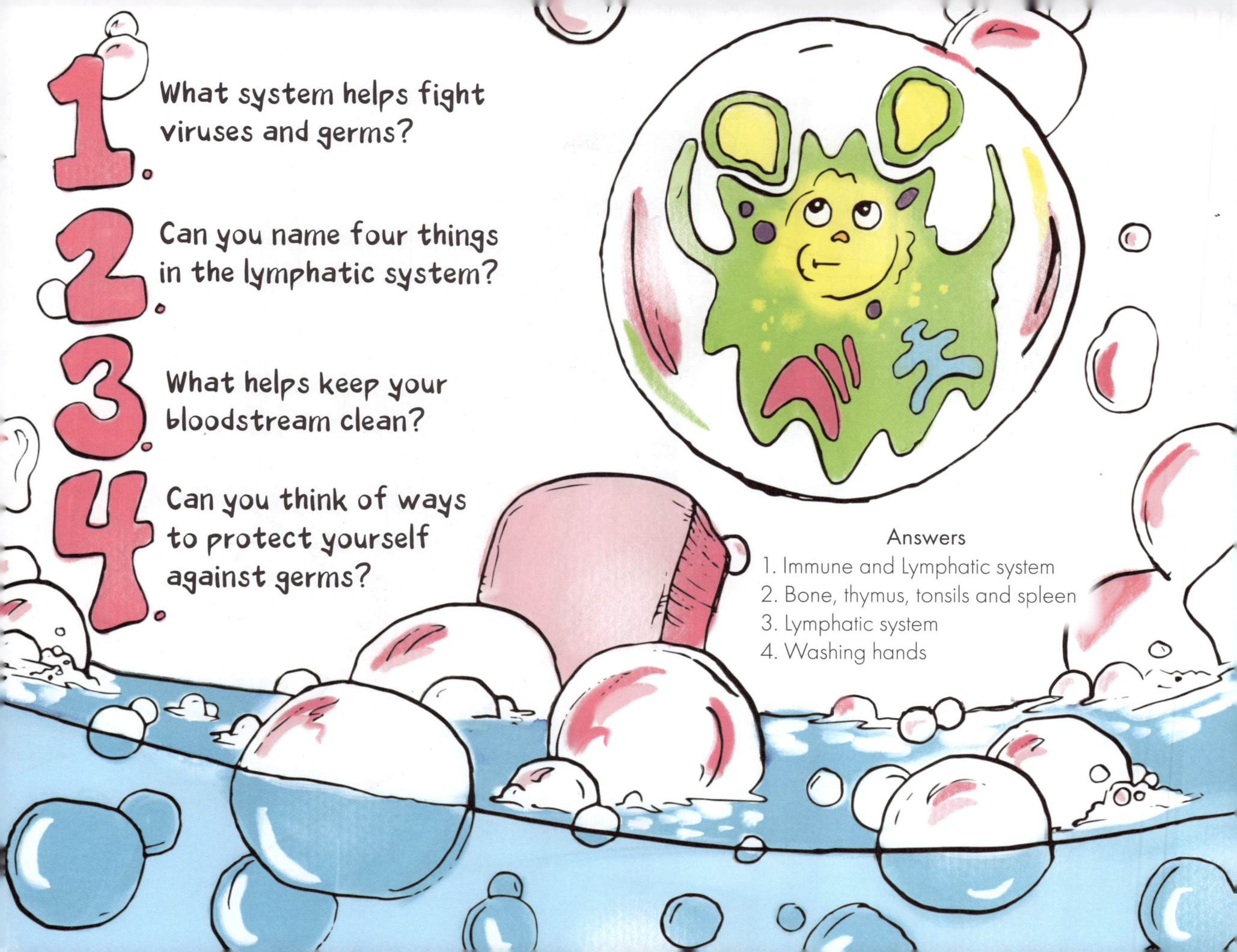

2. Can you name four things in the lymphatic system?

3. What helps keep your bloodstream clean?

4. Can you think of ways to protect yourself against germs?

Answers
1. Immune and Lymphatic system
2. Bone, thymus, tonsils and spleen
3. Lymphatic system
4. Washing hands

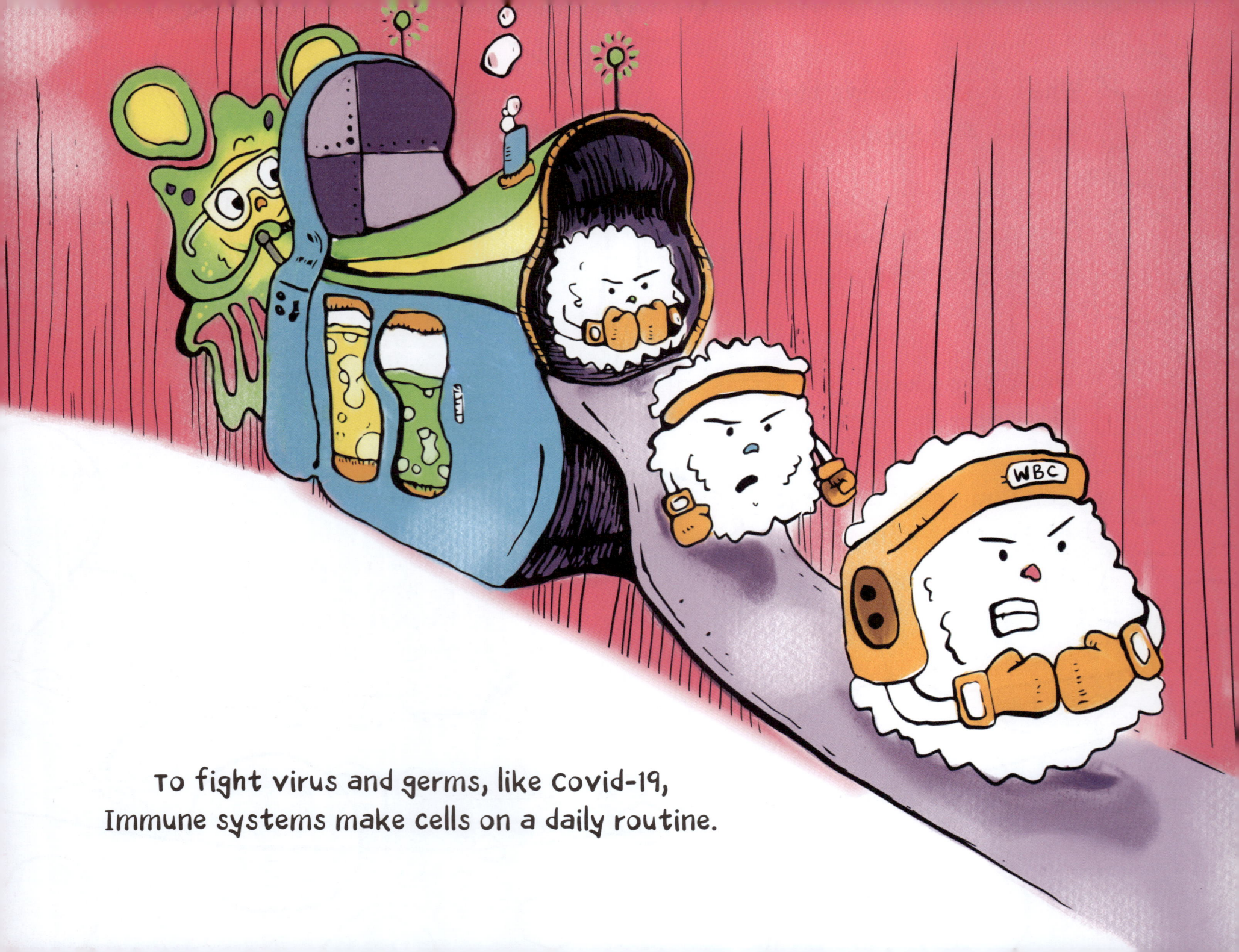

To fight virus and germs, like Covid-19,
Immune systems make cells on a daily routine.

Bones, thymus, the tonsils and even the spleen,

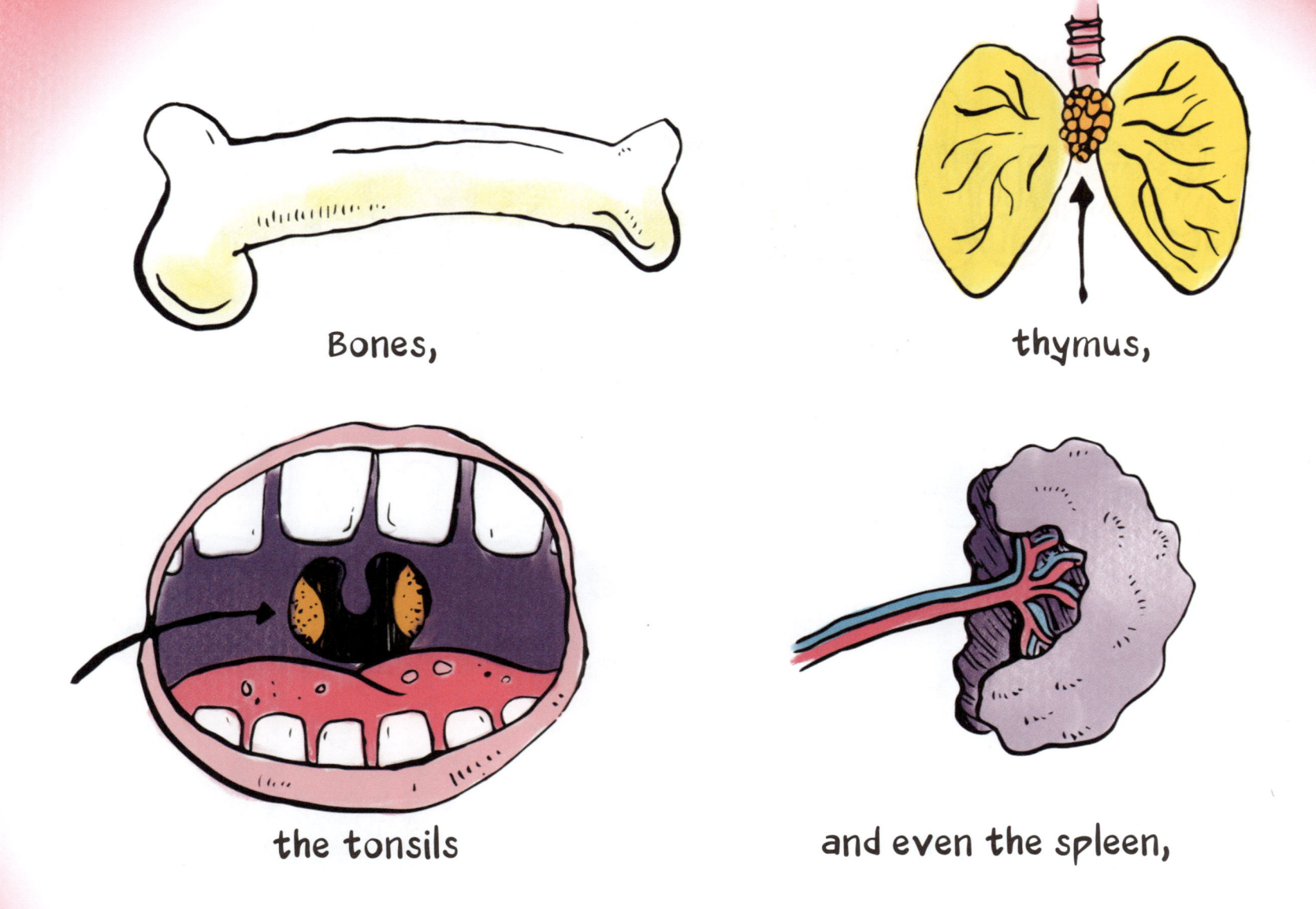

all help to keep your bloodstream clean.

Muscular and Skeletal Systems
(mus-ku-lar)

Shape equals function
so what does that do?
You have skeletal muscles
that's help shaping you.
They grow stronger and bigger
the more you eat food
and protect all your organs
and allow you to move.

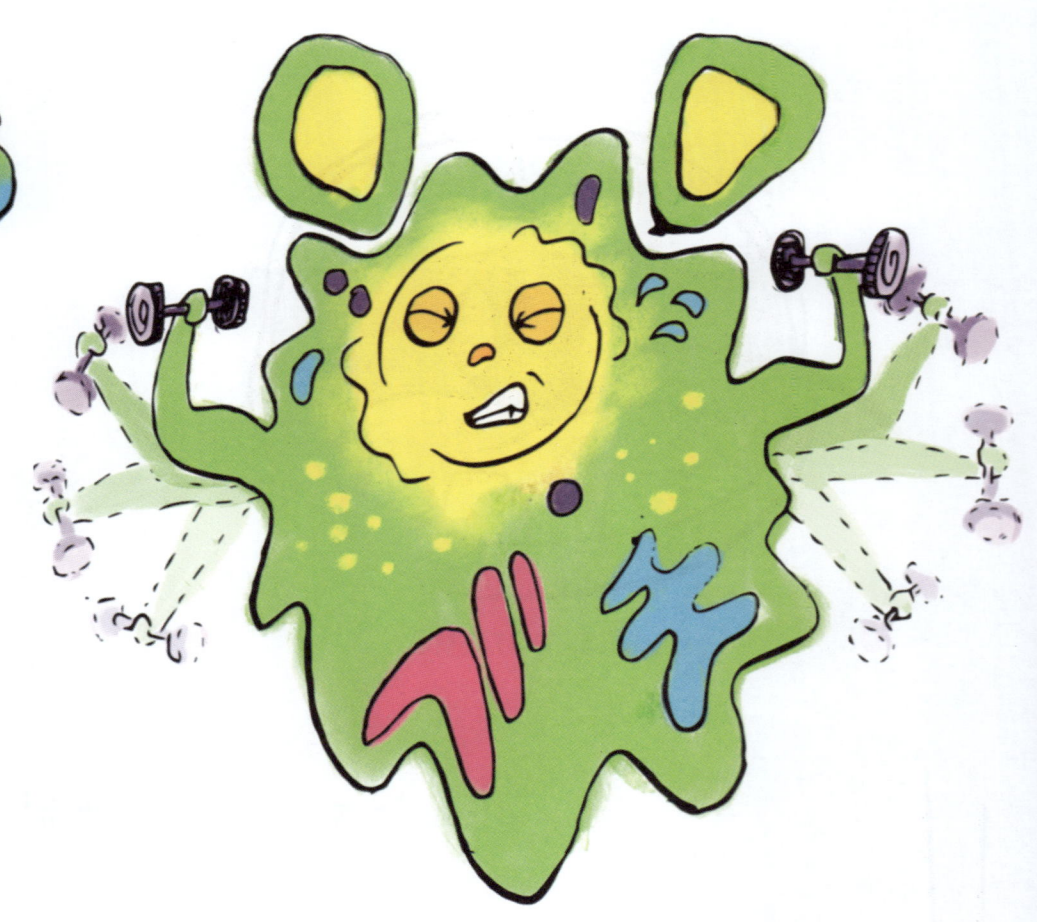

1. How many bones are in the body?

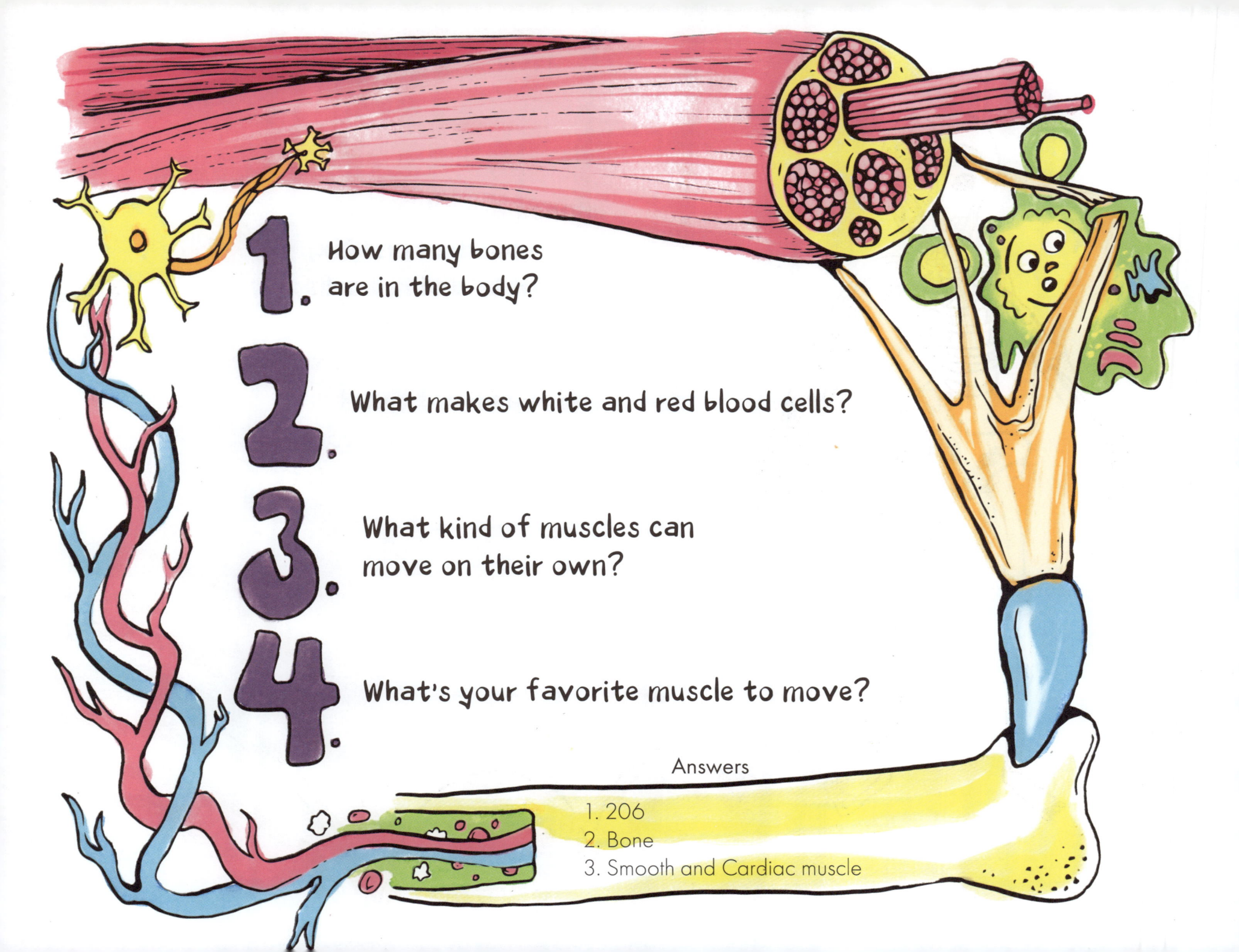

2. What makes white and red blood cells?

3. What kind of muscles can move on their own?

4. What's your favorite muscle to move?

Answers

1. 206
2. Bone
3. Smooth and Cardiac muscle

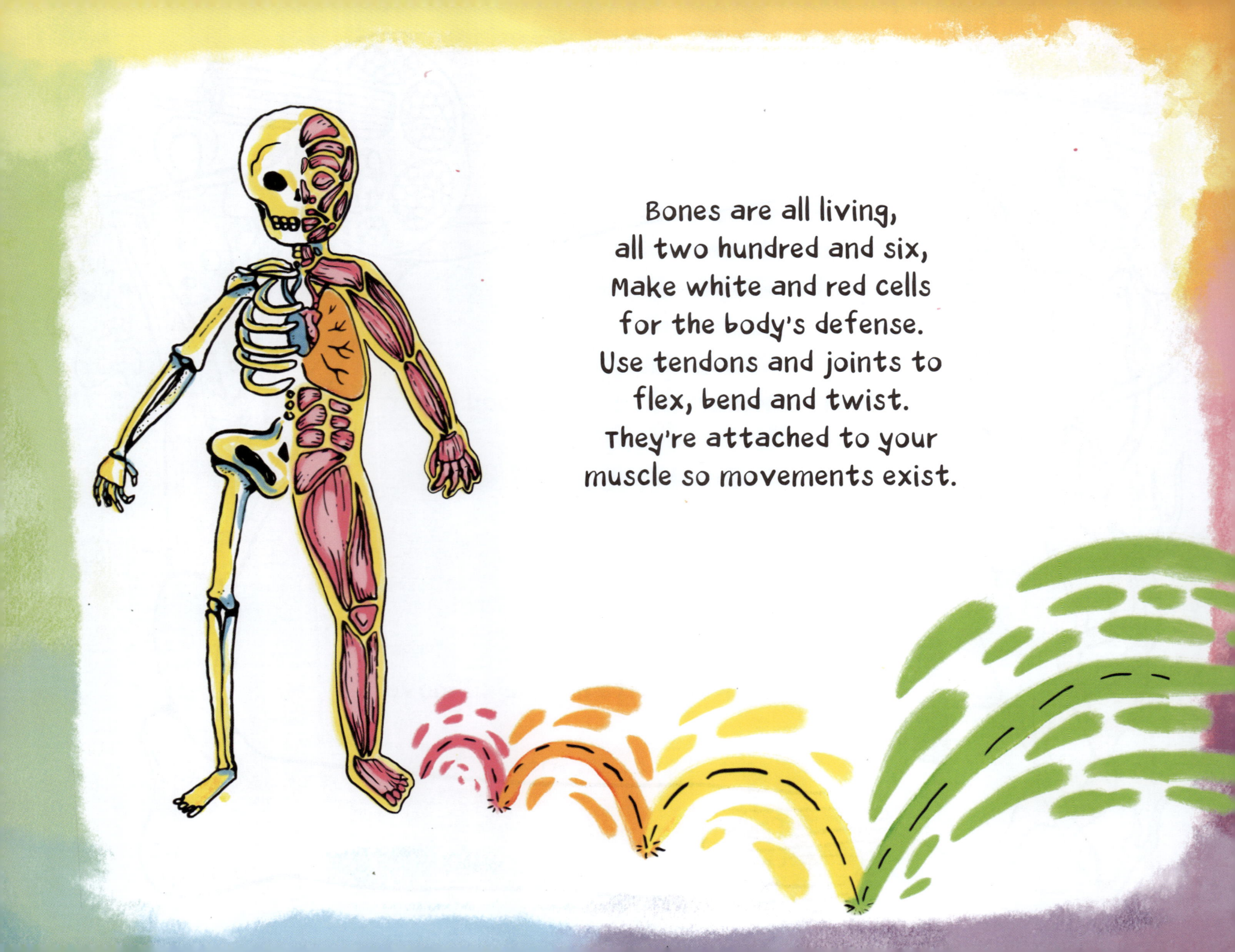

Bones are all living,
all two hundred and six,
Make white and red cells
for the body's defense.
Use tendons and joints to
flex, bend and twist.
They're attached to your
muscle so movements exist.

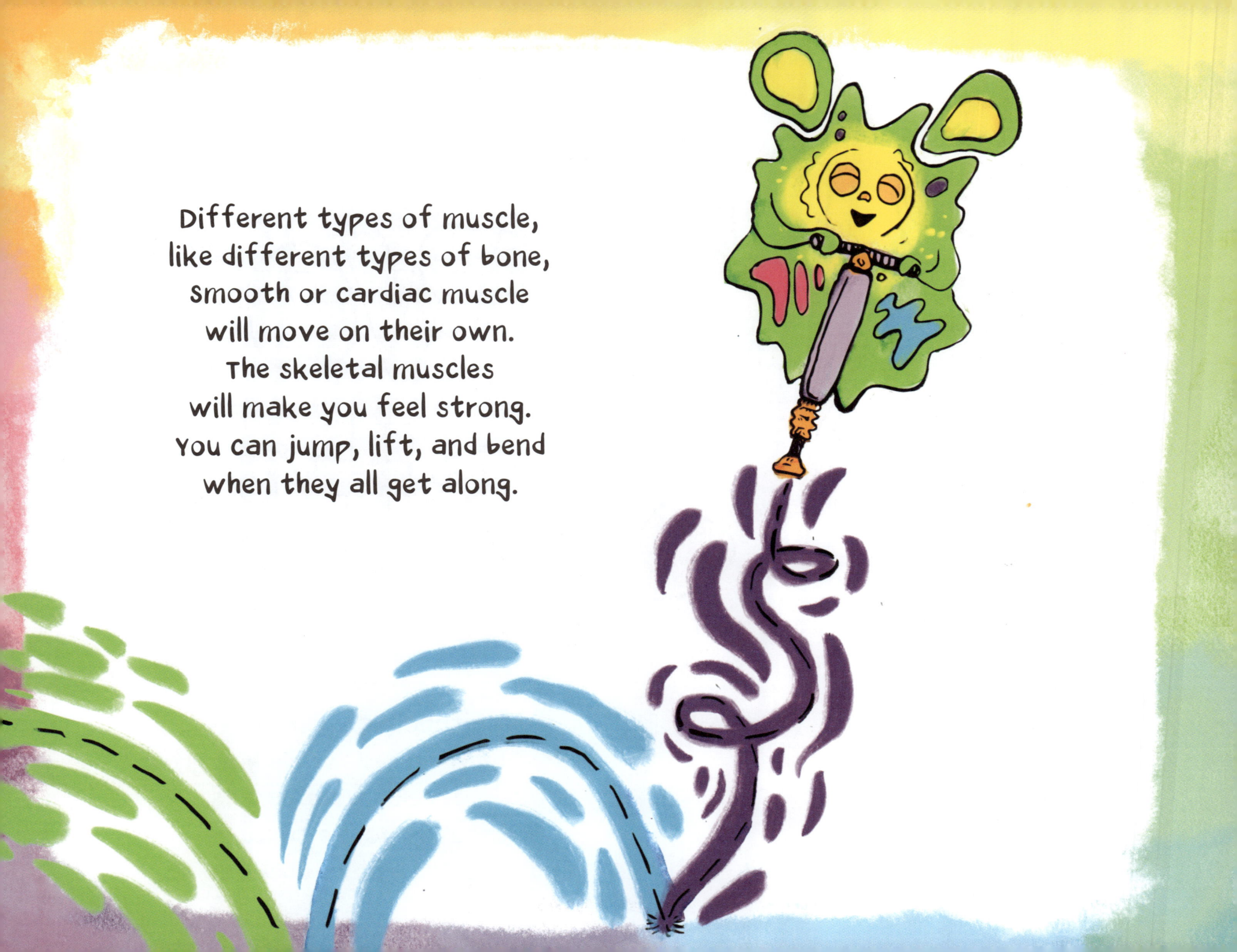

Different types of muscle,
like different types of bone,
smooth or cardiac muscle
will move on their own.
The skeletal muscles
will make you feel strong.
You can jump, lift, and bend
when they all get along.

Nervous System

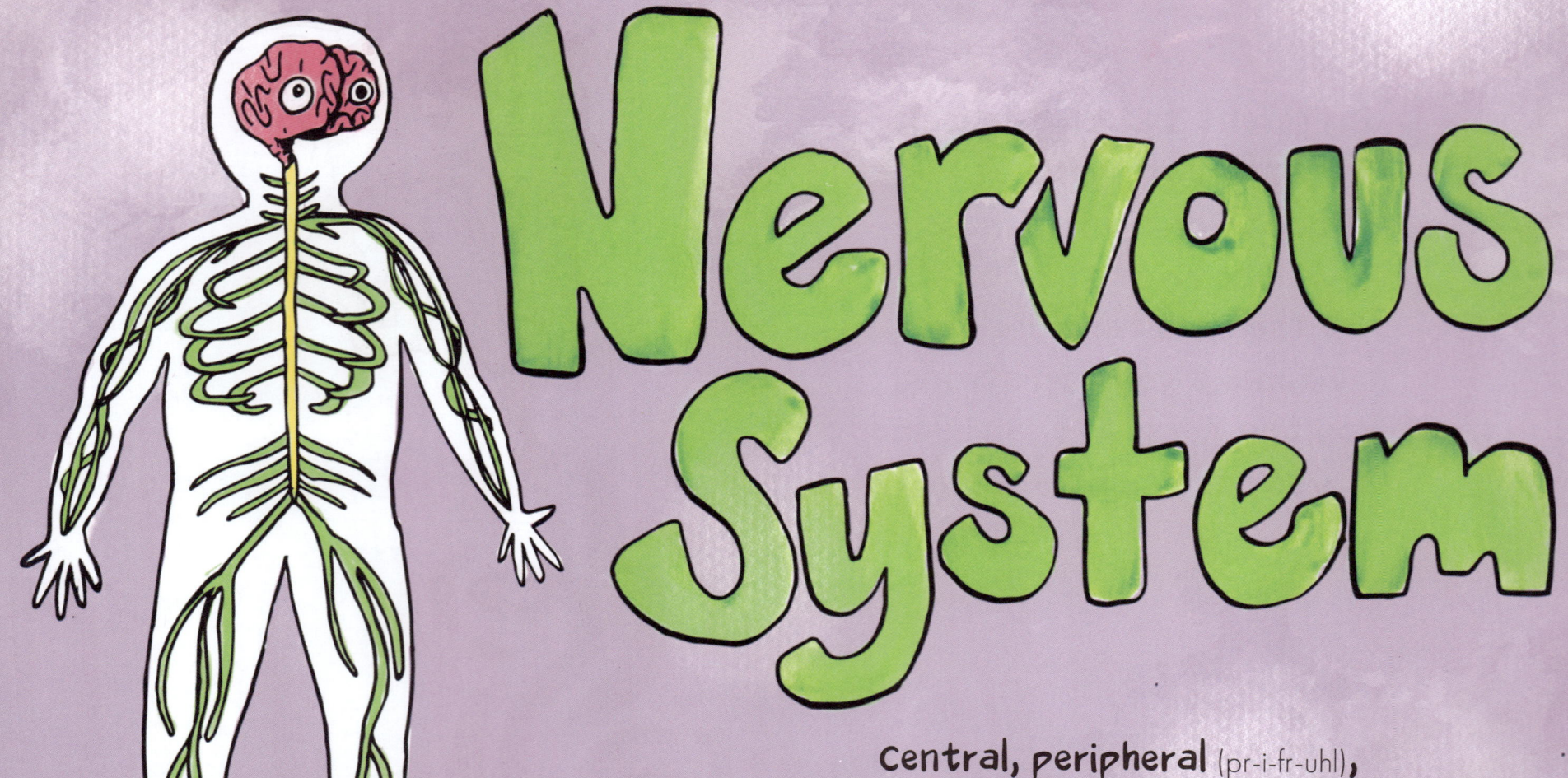

Central, peripheral (pr-i-fr-uhl),
and autonomic (ah-tuh-nah-muhk).
Help your brain cells while you grow,
help develop your senses.
Without it you're senseless
and wouldn't know where to go.

1. What systems make up the nervous system?

2. What organ helps with memory?

3. What are the five senses your brain controls?

4. What's your favorite sense? And why?

Answers
1. Central, peripheral, and autonomic systems
2. Brain
3. Sight, smell, hearing, touch and taste

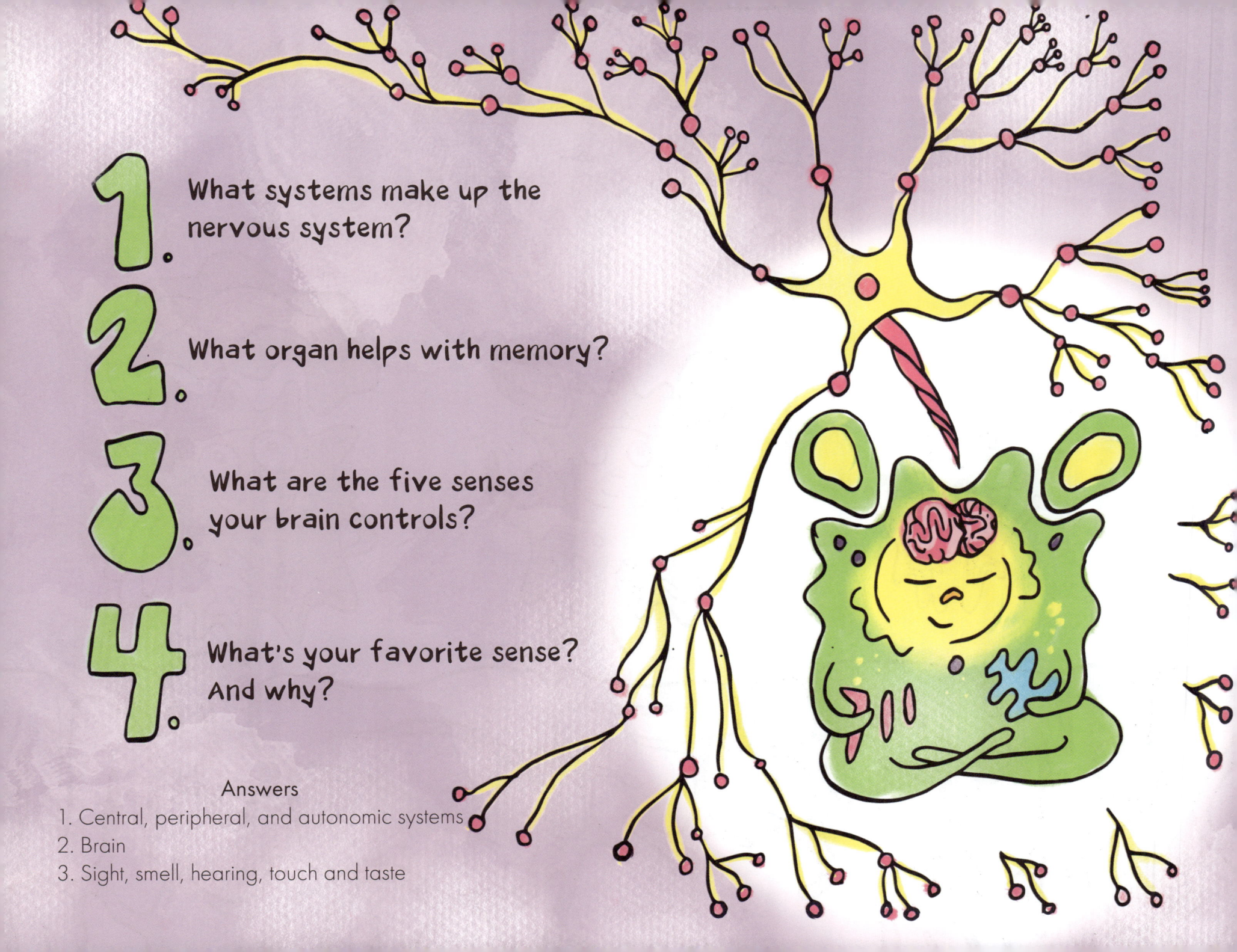

The brain is an organ
with wrinkles and folds.
Stores memory since birth
and as you get old.

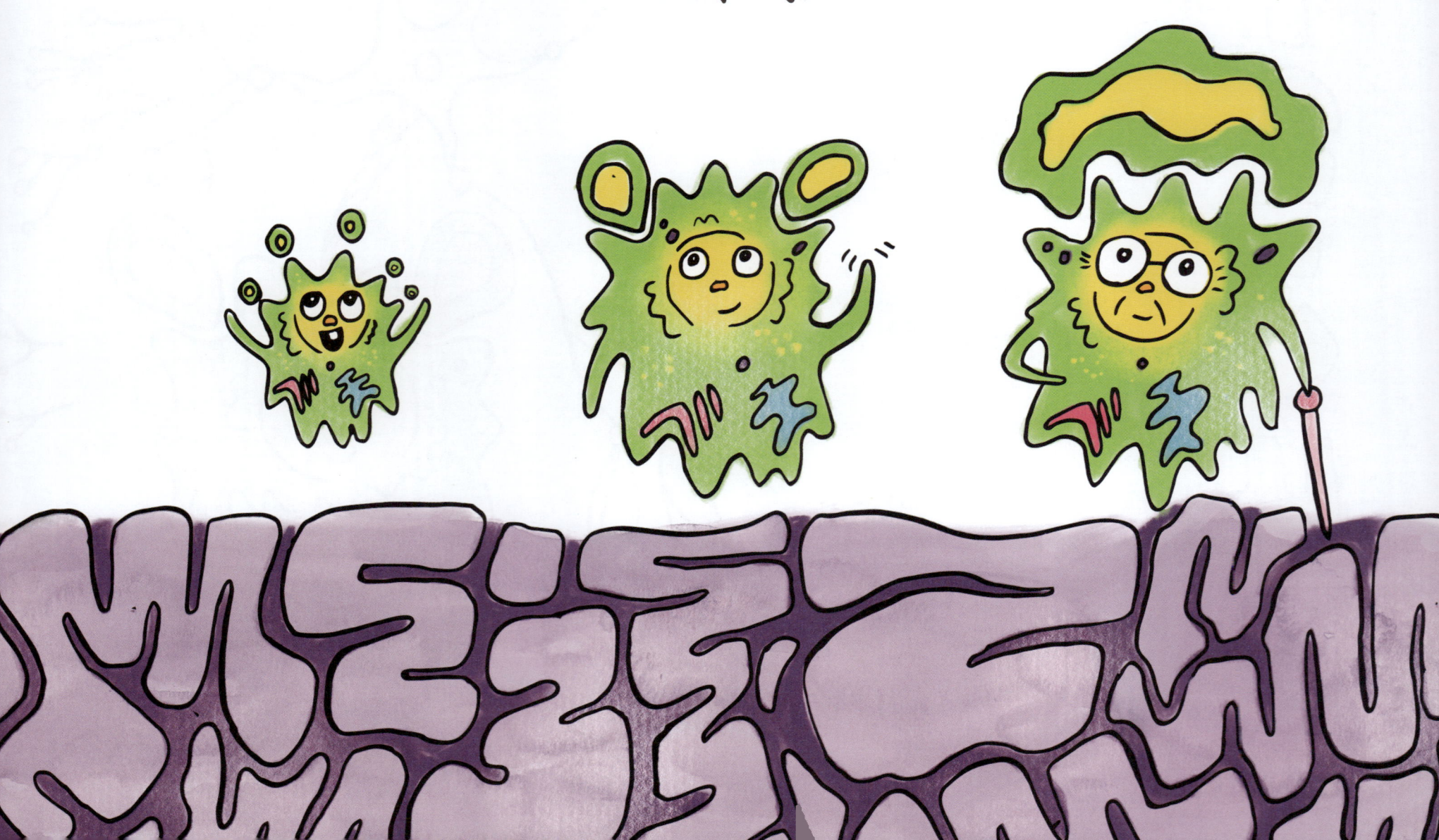

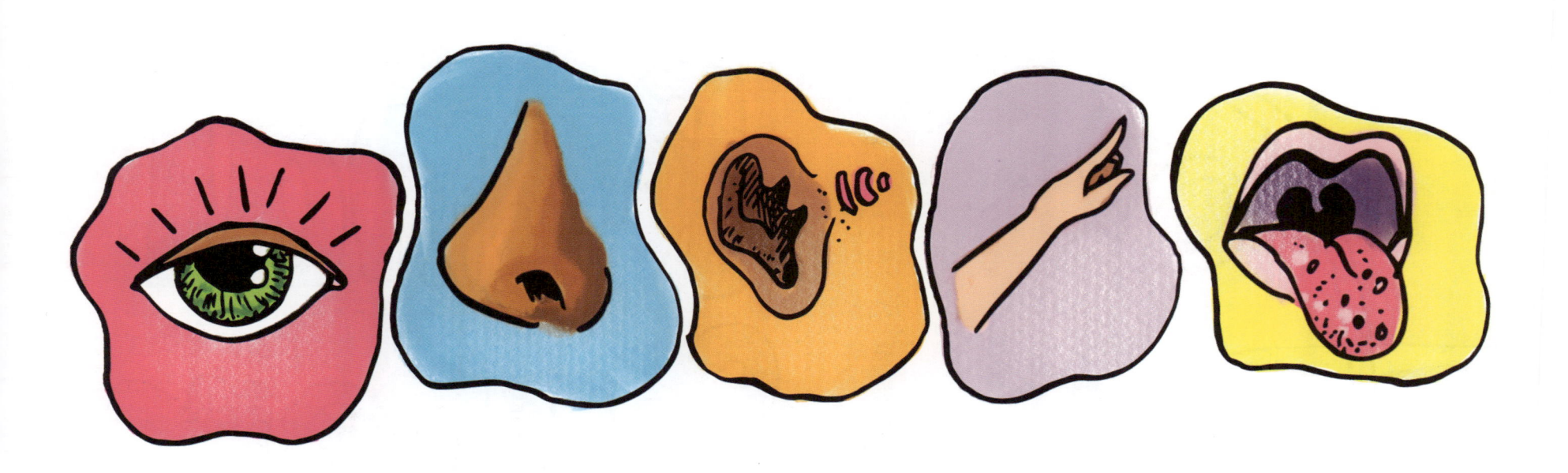

Controls the five senses, so we do not waste,
sight, smell, or sound, touch, nor our taste.
It uses these senses, to think and react,
Move and keep balance, defend or attack.

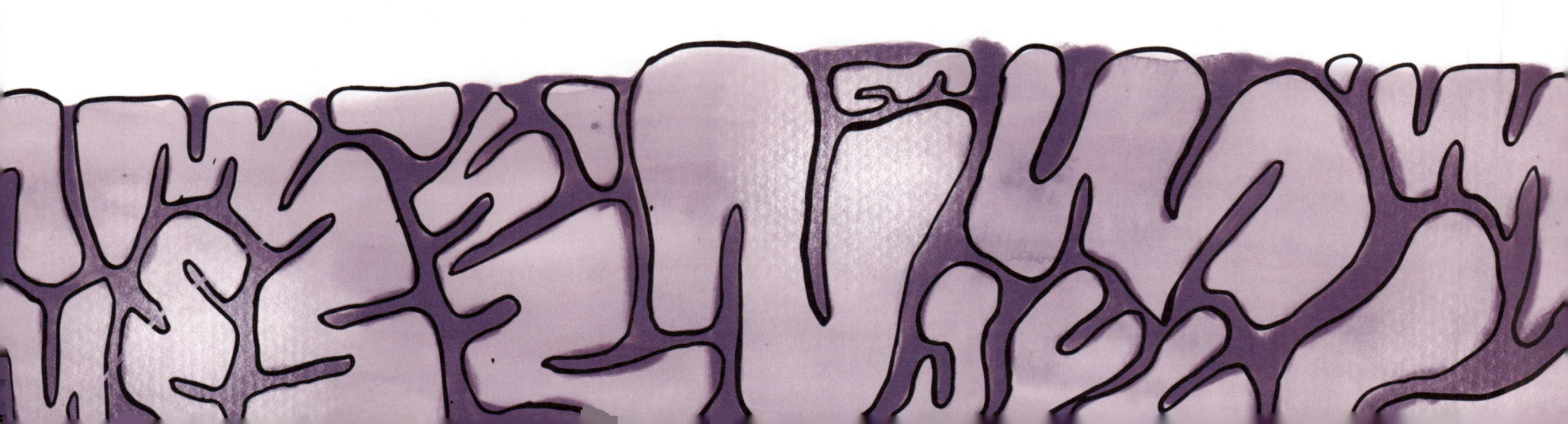

Renal System

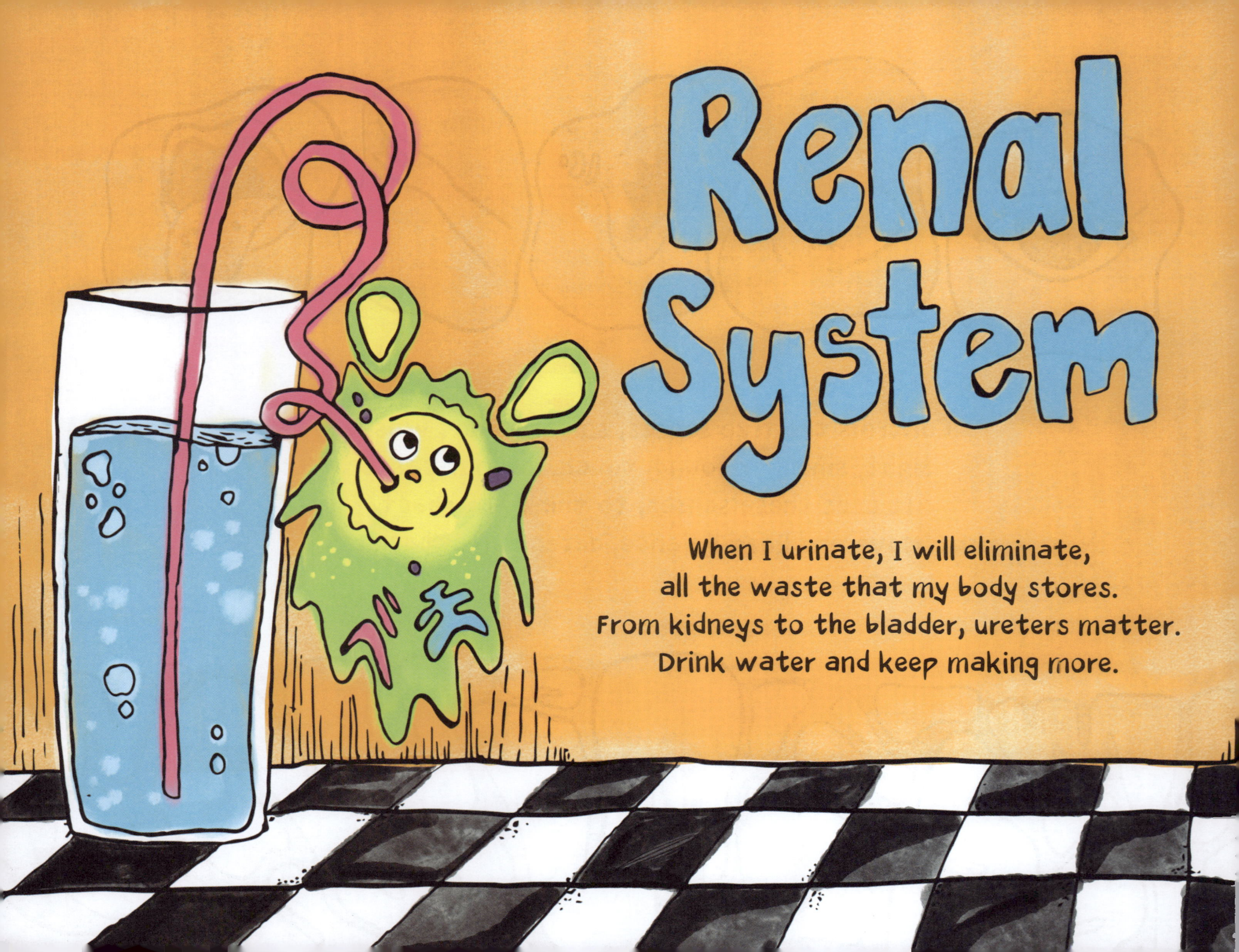

When I urinate, I will eliminate,
all the waste that my body stores.
From kidneys to the bladder, ureters matter.
Drink water and keep making more.

1. What helps make urine?

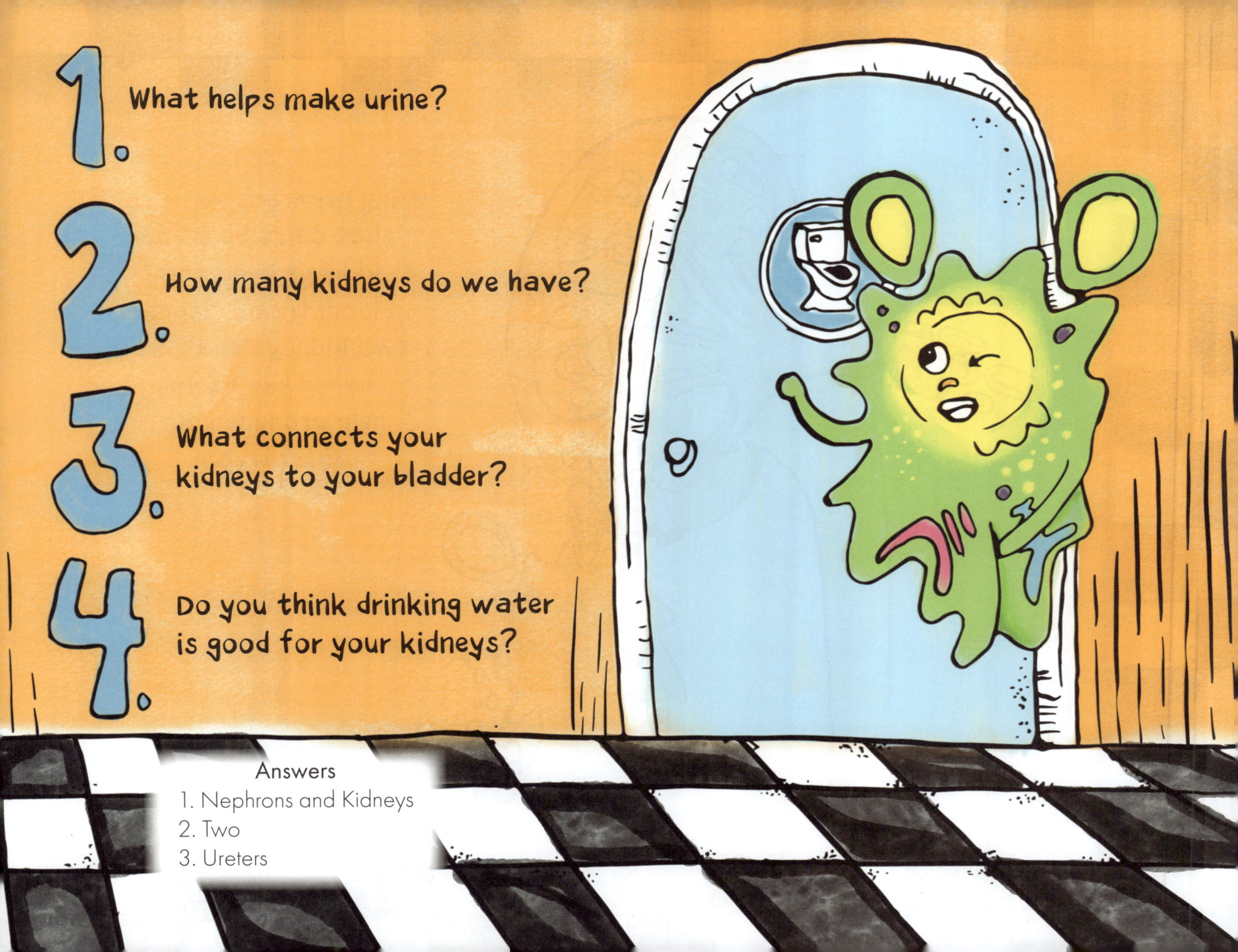

2. How many kidneys do we have?

3. What connects your kidneys to your bladder?

4. Do you think drinking water is good for your kidneys?

Answers
1. Nephrons and Kidneys
2. Two
3. Ureters

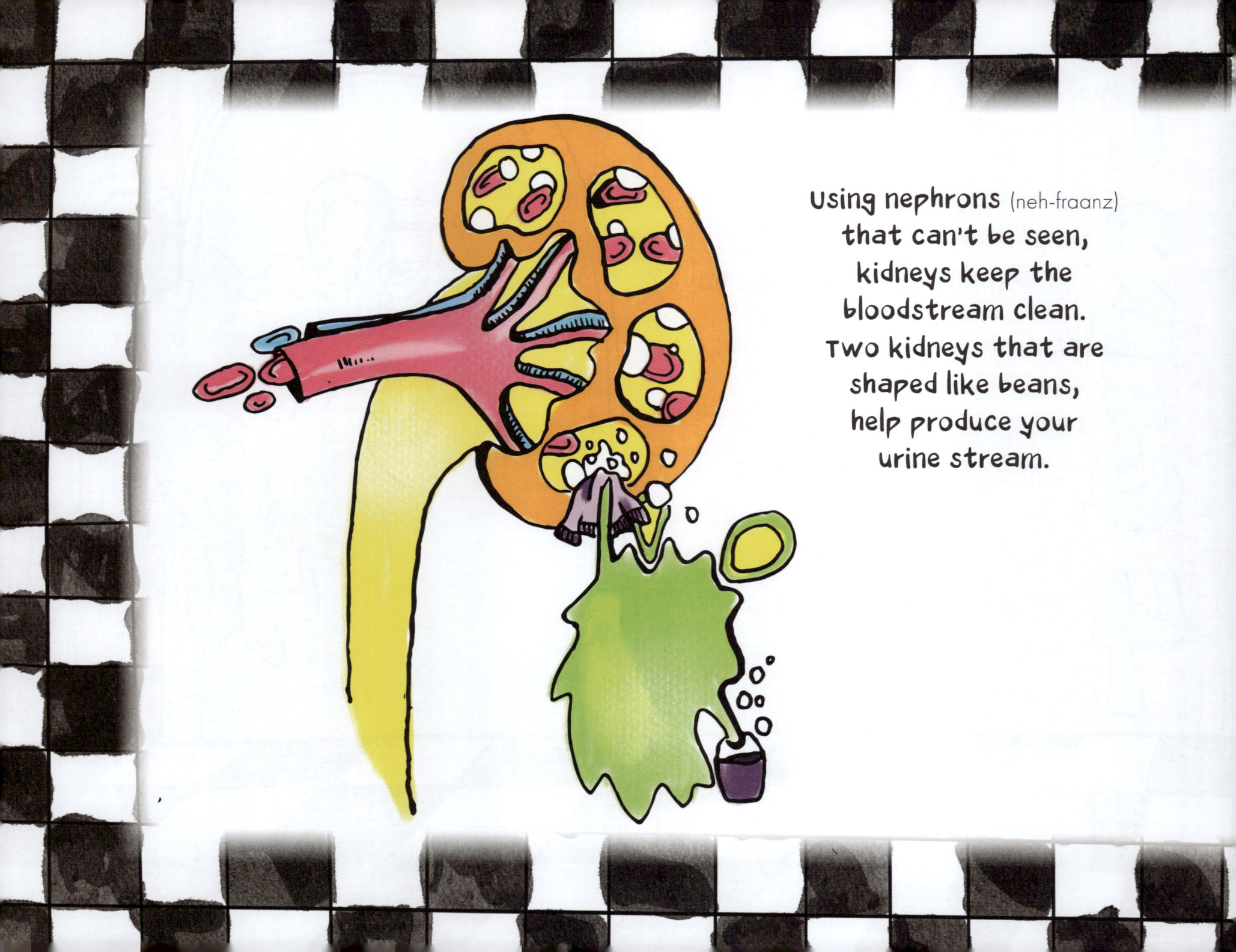

Using nephrons (neh-fraanz) that can't be seen, kidneys keep the bloodstream clean. Two kidneys that are shaped like beans, help produce your urine stream.

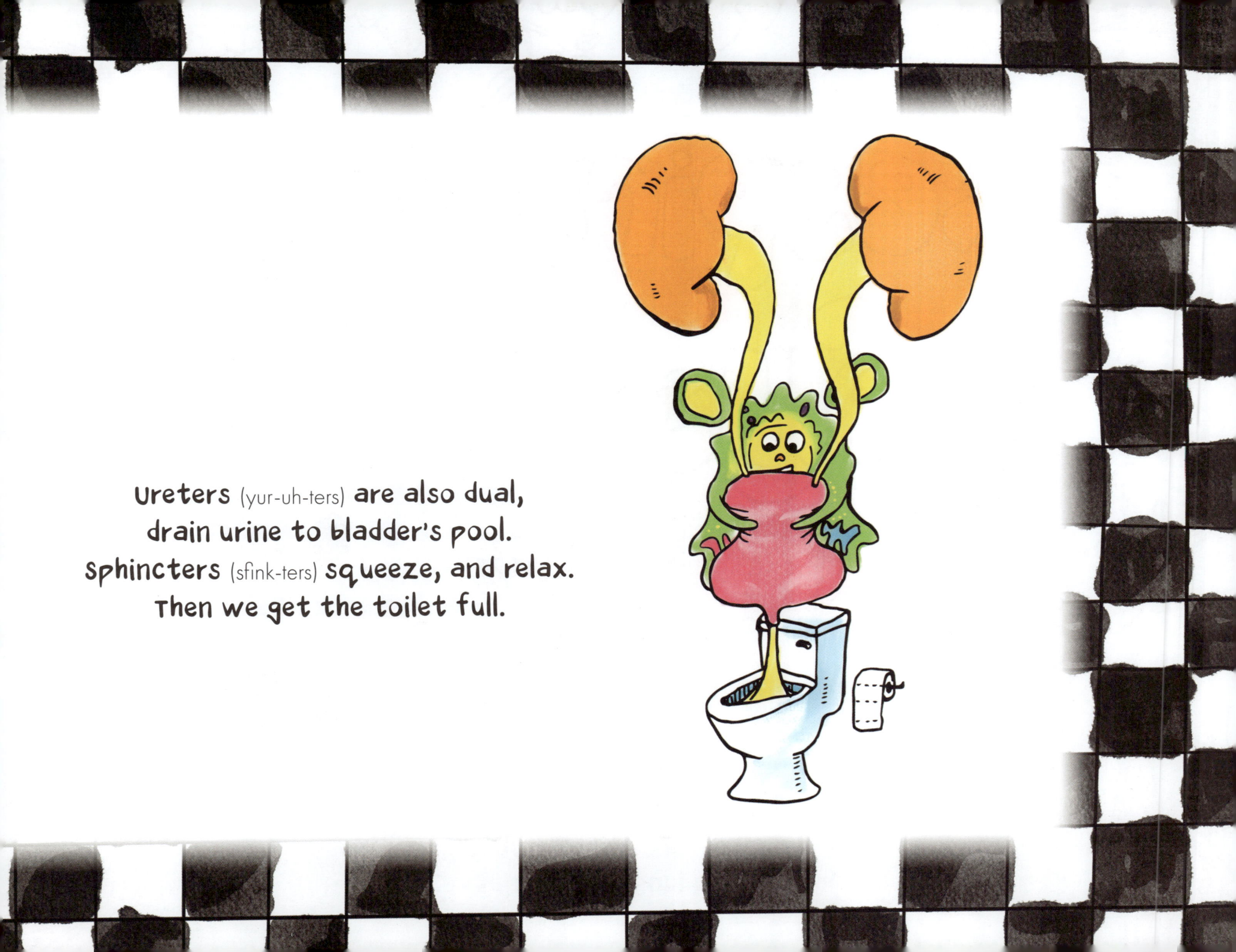

Ureters (yur-uh-ters) are also dual,
drain urine to bladder's pool.
Sphincters (sfink-ters) squeeze, and relax.
Then we get the toilet full.

Respiratory System
(reh-spr-uh-taw-ree)

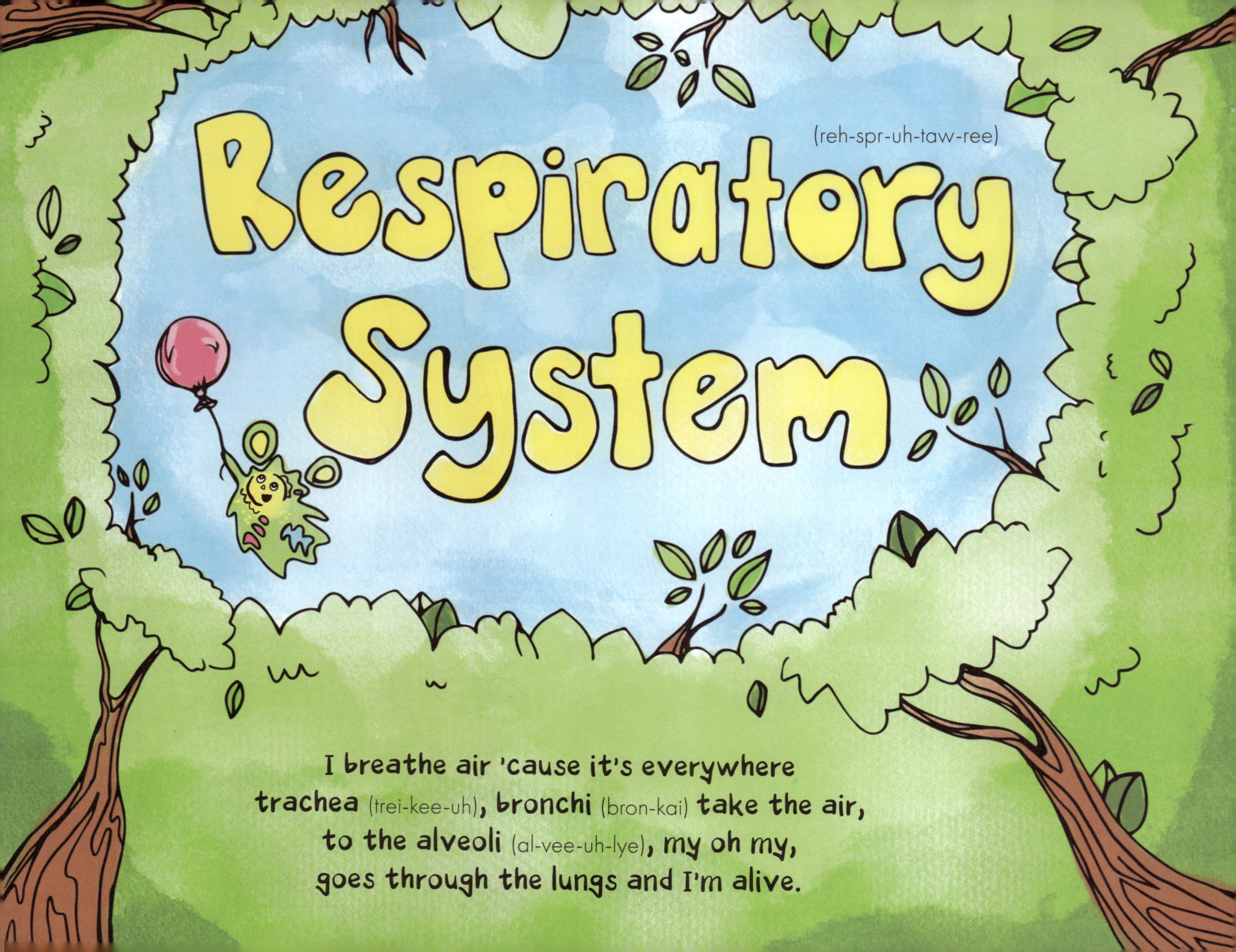

I breathe air 'cause it's everywhere
trachea (trei-kee-uh), bronchi (bron-kai) take the air,
to the alveoli (al-vee-uh-lye), my oh my,
goes through the lungs and I'm alive.

1. What muscle does the lung use to breath?

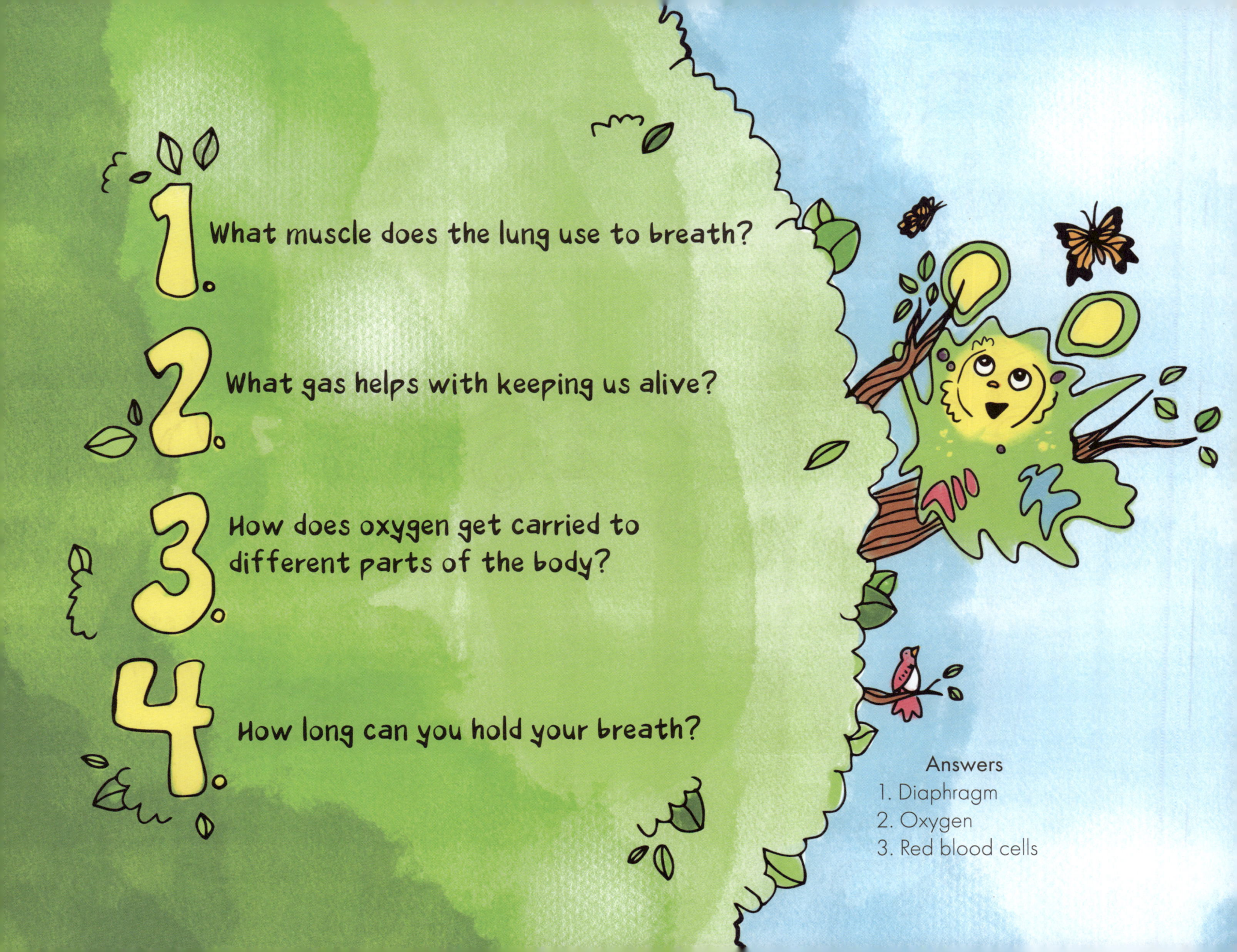

2. What gas helps with keeping us alive?

3. How does oxygen get carried to different parts of the body?

4. How long can you hold your breath?

Answers
1. Diaphragm
2. Oxygen
3. Red blood cells

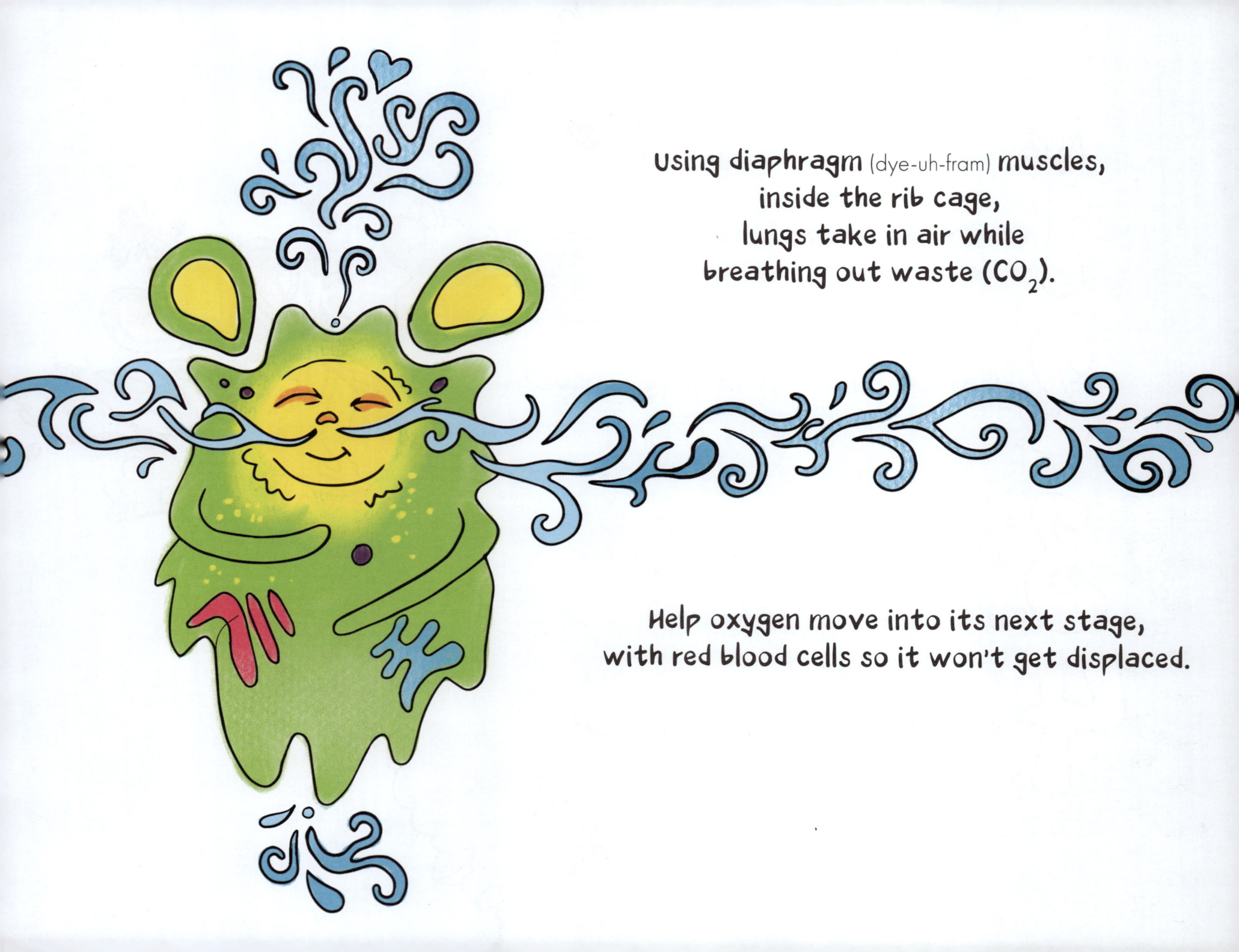

Using diaphragm (dye-uh-fram) muscles, inside the rib cage, lungs take in air while breathing out waste (CO_2).

Help oxygen move into its next stage, with red blood cells so it won't get displaced.

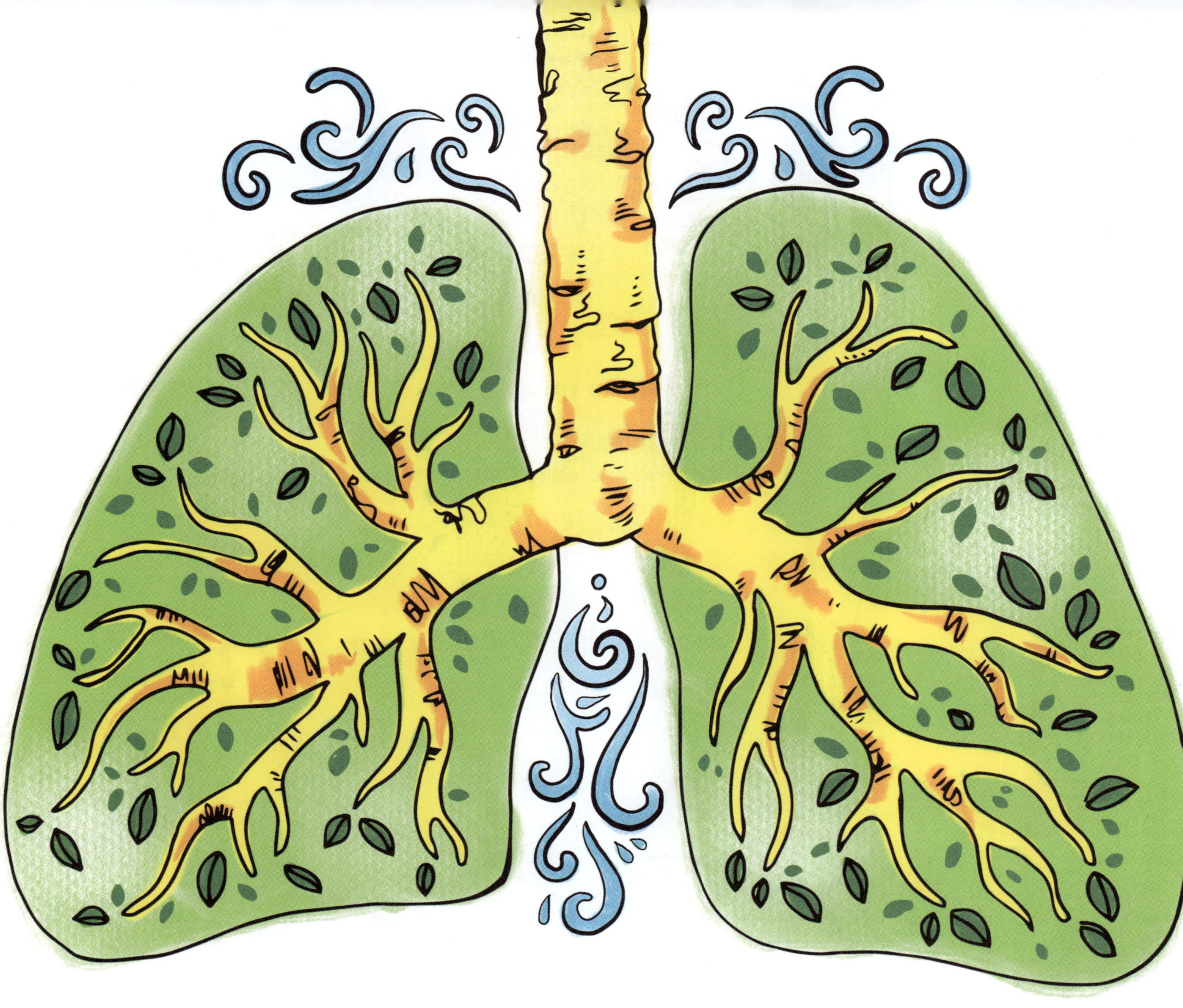

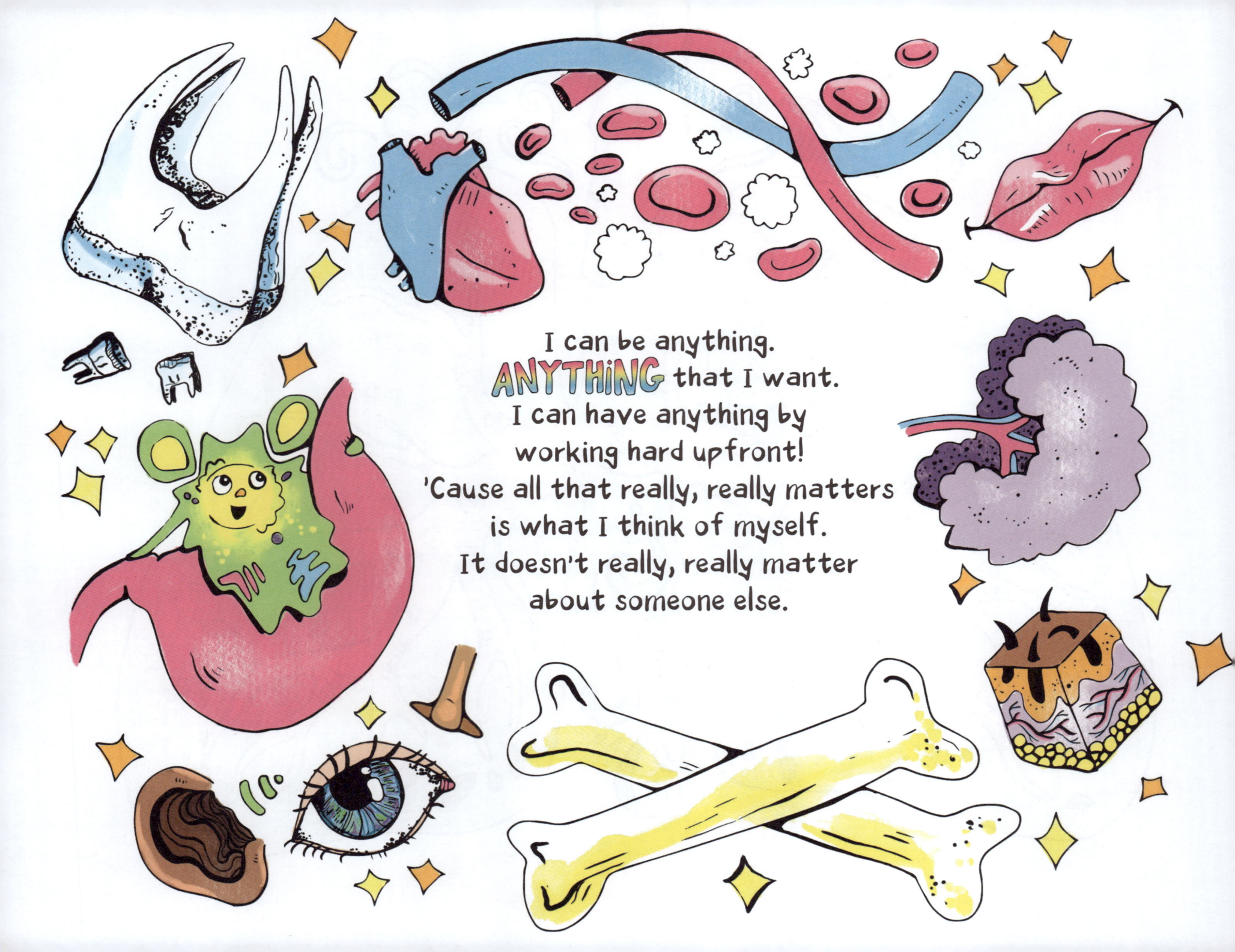

I can be anything. **ANYTHING** that I want.
I can have anything by working hard upfront!
'Cause all that really, really matters is what I think of myself.
It doesn't really, really matter about someone else.

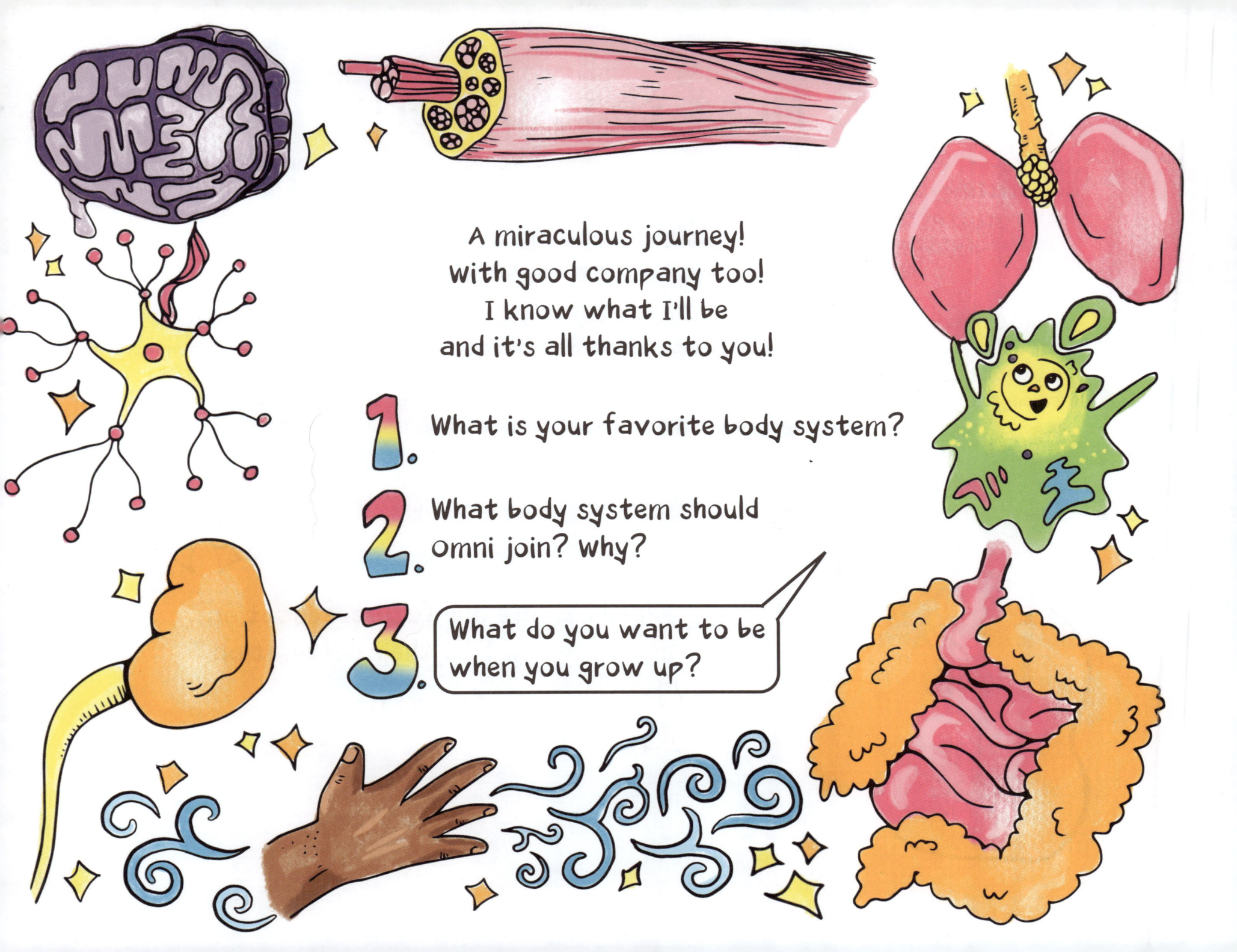

A miraculous journey!
with good company too!
I know what I'll be
and it's all thanks to you!

1. What is your favorite body system?

2. What body system should Omni join? why?

3. What do you want to be when you grow up?

✦ Meet the Author!

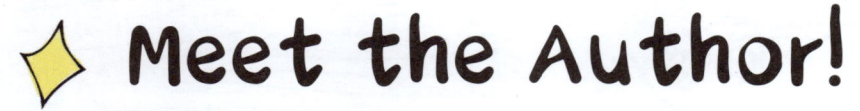

Dr. Steven Patton was born in Chicago, Illinois, and raised in Covert, Michigan. He earned a bachelor's degree in biology with a minor in chemistry from Kentucky State University and his medical degree from the University of Pikeville - Kentucky College of Osteopathic Medicine. He completed his family medicine residency at Community Westview Hospital in Indianapolis, Indiana. He is board certified in family medicine and is a member of the American Osteopathic Association.

In 2021, he was named medical director for community outreach. In this role he participates in educational health programs and events with a focus on addressing health equity in underserved areas. Dr. Patton also collaborates with the Institute for Health Equity, a part of Norton Healthcare, to strengthen community relations and access to care to improve health equity statistics. He enjoys reading, learning different styles of martial arts and finding fun ways in educating the community.

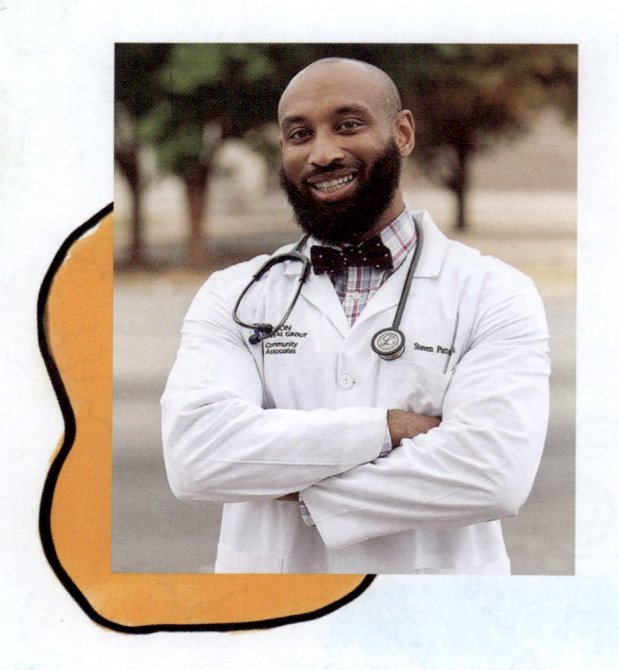

"Children are our future. Education helps them get to their destination."

- Dr. Steven Patton

CASCADE VALLEY CO

Welcome to "Cascade Valley Cocktails: PNW locally crafted libations" - a celebration of the vibrant flavors and rich traditions found in the heart of the Pacific Northwest. Situated amidst the breathtaking landscapes of Enumclaw, Buckley, Puyallup, and Sumner, you'll discover the fertile fields and artisanal enterprises that define our local communites.

In this delightful collection of farm-to-table cocktails, we invite you to embark on a journey through the lush valleys and rolling hills of Pierce County. Here, the values of sustainability and the love for quality craftsmanship come together harmoniously. Each recipe in this book is a testament to the abundant harvests and culinary brilliance that thrive within our region, featuring the finest ingredients sourced directly from our local farms and producers.

While some recipes showcase the crisp rhubarb from our area's farms, others highlight the incredible produce and unmatched creativity of our local businesses. As you embark on this flavorful expedition, we encourage you to savor each sip, appreciating the stories of community, sustainability, and the unwavering connection between our land and those who nurture it.

Brought to you by the Sumner Main Street Association to celebrate their Rhubarb Days festival and Reyna Robyn Photography.

TABLE OF CONTENTS

Prosecco Float..pg. 4
Valley Social Wine Bar, Sumner

Electric Spro Martini..pg. 6
Electric Coffee House, Sumner

Electric Rhubarb Margarita..pg. 8
Electric Coffee House, Sumner

Rhubarb Seltzer..pg. 10
Griffin Brewing Co, Enumclaw

Raspberries & Cream Margarita...pg. 12
Main Street Bistro, Buckley

The Genevieve Cocktail...pg. 14
Simple Goodness Sisters, Wilkeson

Limoncello Martini..pg. 16
Sorci's Italian Cafe, Sumner

Berry Cobbler...pg. 18
The Bistro at Windmill Gardens, Sumner

Hot Summer...pg. 20
The Bistro at Windmill Gardens, Sumner

TABLE OF CONTENTS

Fierce County Ginger Rye..pg. 22
Fierce County Cider, Puyallup

Inta Pink..pg. 24
Inta Vintage, Sumner

Strawberry Rhubarb Lemonade..pg. 26
Knutson Farms, Sumner

Ginger Margarita..pg. 28
Locale Plants, Sumner

Dirty Martini..pg. 30
Bomb Charcuterie, Sumner

Jungle Cat..pg. 32
Township 20, Sumner

Rhapple Rhardamom Sprit..pg. 34
Township 20, Sumner

A Little Ginger on Your Mind Americano..pg. 36
Untamed Coffee, Sumner

Ginger Drops & What the Ginger Muddy Soda..pg. 37 & 38
Untamed Coffee, Sumner

Smootharita..pg. 40
Eternal Soul Bowl, Sumner

Strawberry Mojito..pg. 42
Reyna Robyn Photography, Bonney Lake

PROSECCO FLOAT
Valley Social Wine Bar

A neighborhood wine bar featuring small bites, shared plates, great wine, and gourmet gelato, in a contemporary inviting atmosphere. Located on main street in Sumner, the perfect place to sit back, relax and enjoy a glass or two!

Recipe

- Mini scoop of strawberry rhubarb gelato (available in June or try with a flavor of your choice)
- Chilled Prosecco

Directions

1. Head to Valley Social Wine Bar and get gelato and a bottle of prosecco to-go!
2. Chill the prosecco and a coupe glass
3. Put a mini scoop of gelato in the chilled coupe glass, top with prosecco, ENJOY!

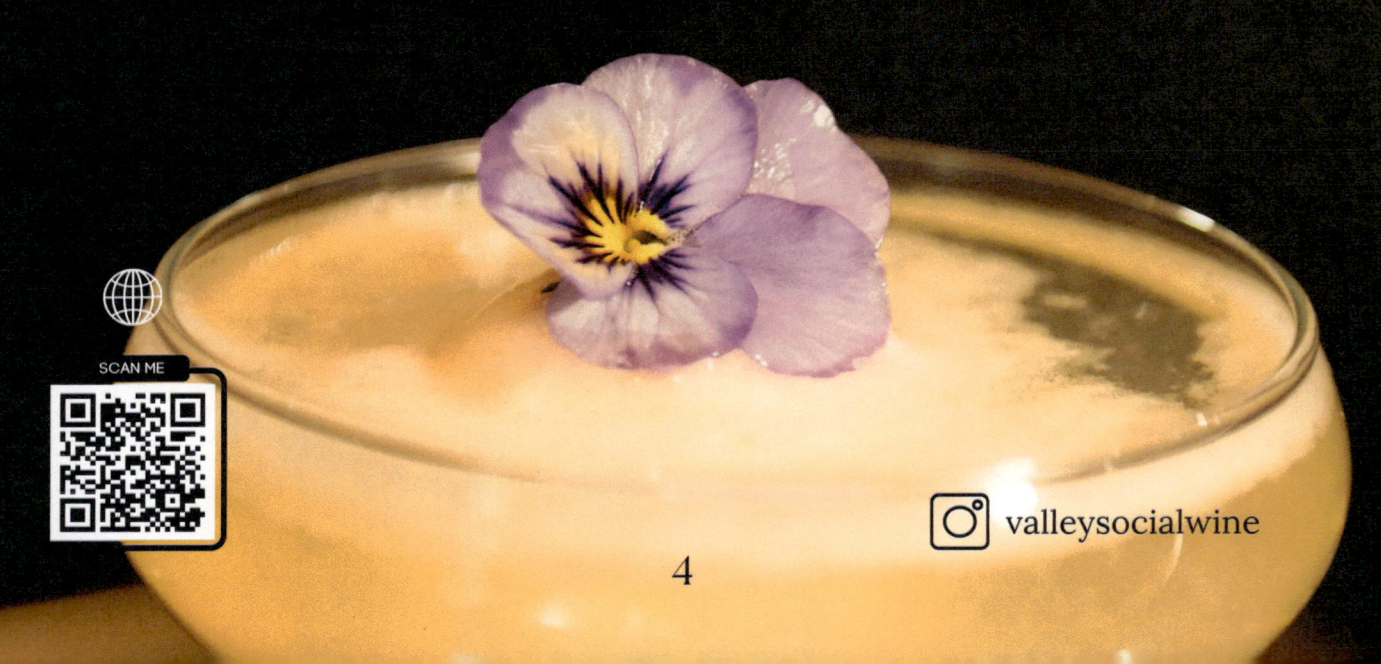

valleysocialwine

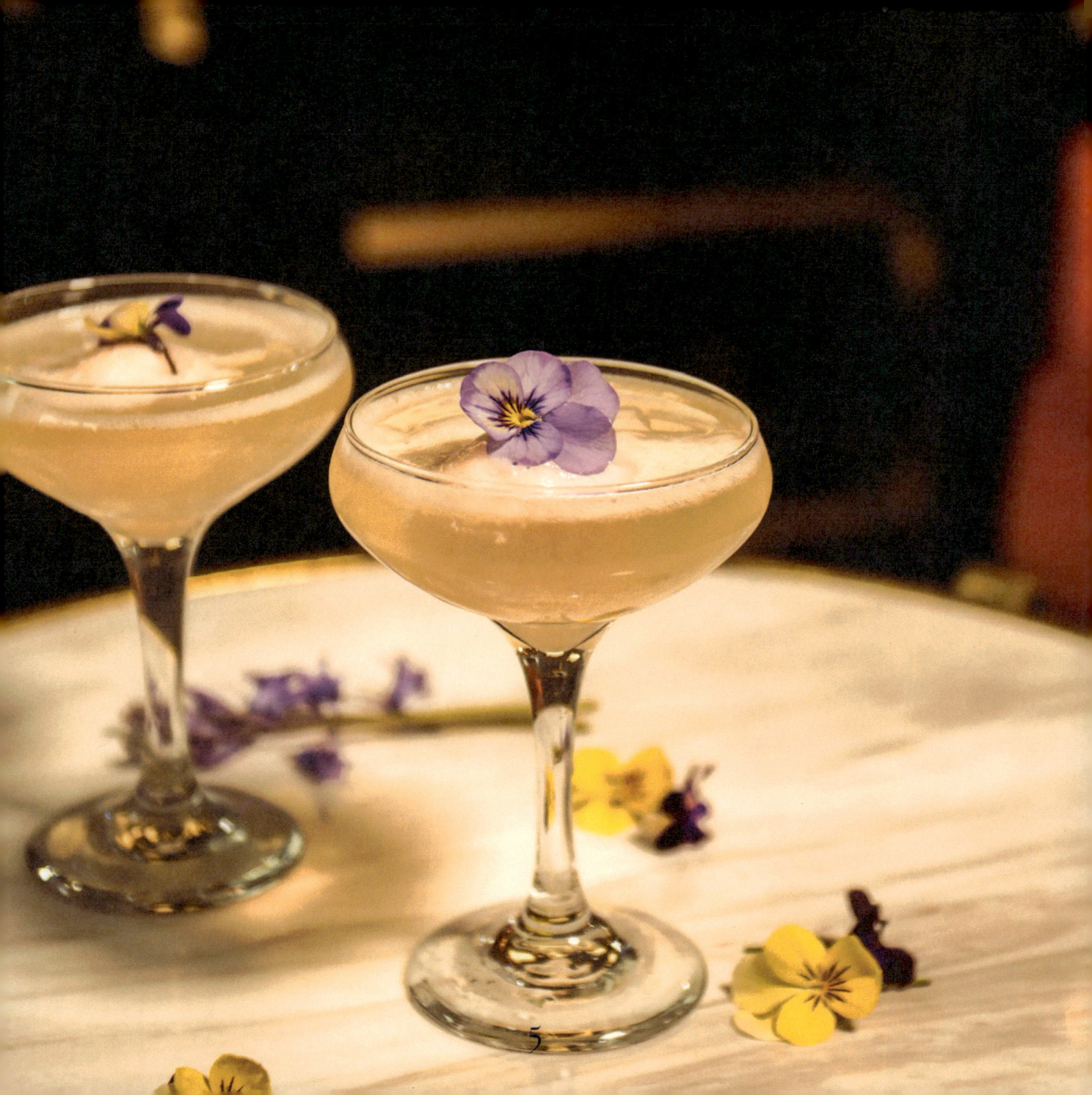

ELECTRIC SPRO MARTINI
Electric Coffee House

Recipe

2oz Tequila
1oz Kahlúa
1oz Baileys
1oz Espresso
1/2 oz simple syrup
1 cup of ice
3 Espresso Beans

Directions

1. Gather ingredients
2. Combine 1 oz of Baileys, 1 ounce of Kahlúa, and 2 oz of tequila in shaker
3. Pull your espresso shot
4. Add 1 oz of espresso to shaker, along with 1/2 oz of simple syrup
5. Add 1 cup of ice cubes to shaker
6. Shake until frothy
7. Pour in a glass and garnish with 3 espresso beans

If you're looking for an aesthetic but welcoming spot to enjoy something tasty, then you've come to the right place. Entrées, craft cocktails, desserts, and of course, coffee, await at your new favorite Sumner hangout:
Electric Coffee House.

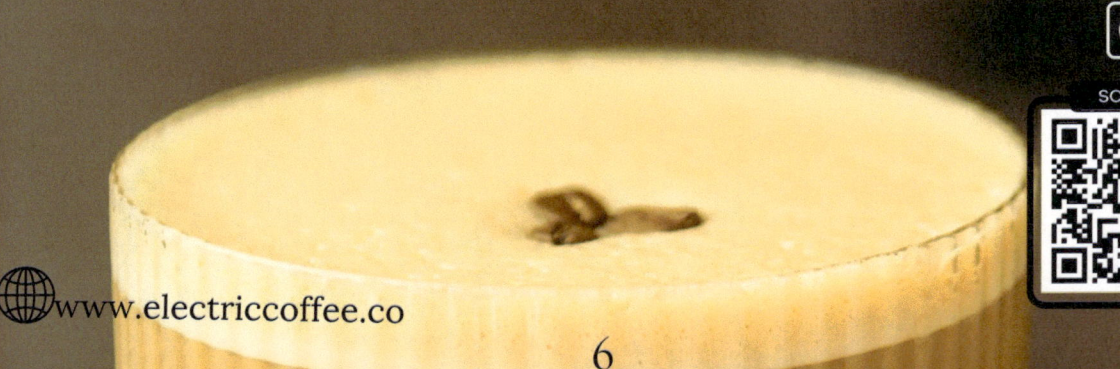

www.electriccoffee.co

SCAN ME

7

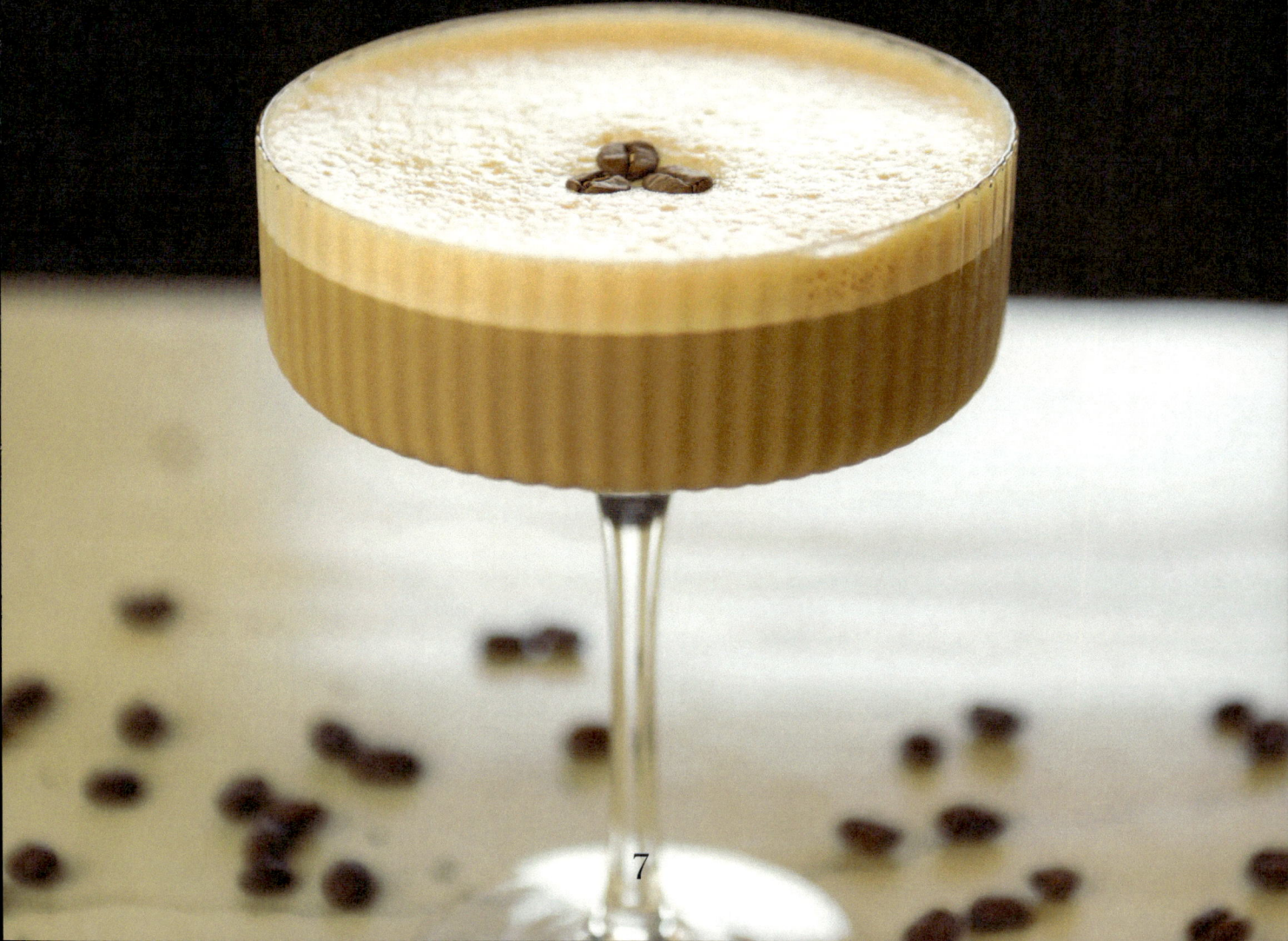

ELECTRIC RHUBARB MARGARITA
Electric Coffee House

Recipe

1oz Simple Goodness Sisters Rhubarb Vanilla Bean Syrup
1 oz lime juice
2oz tequila
1 cup of ice
1 ice cube

Directions

1. Add Simple Goodness Sisters Rhubarb Vanilla Bean Syrup, lime juice, tequila, and 1 cup of ice to shaker
2. Shake well
3. Add an ice cube to glass
4. Pour shaken cocktail on top of ice cube
5. Garnish with fruit (optional)

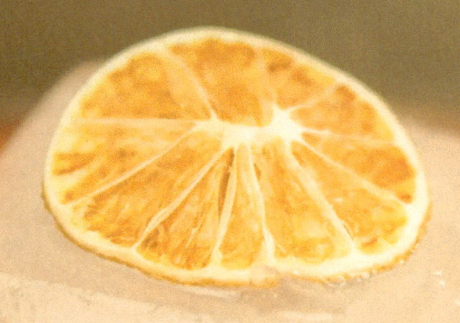

www.electriccoffee.co

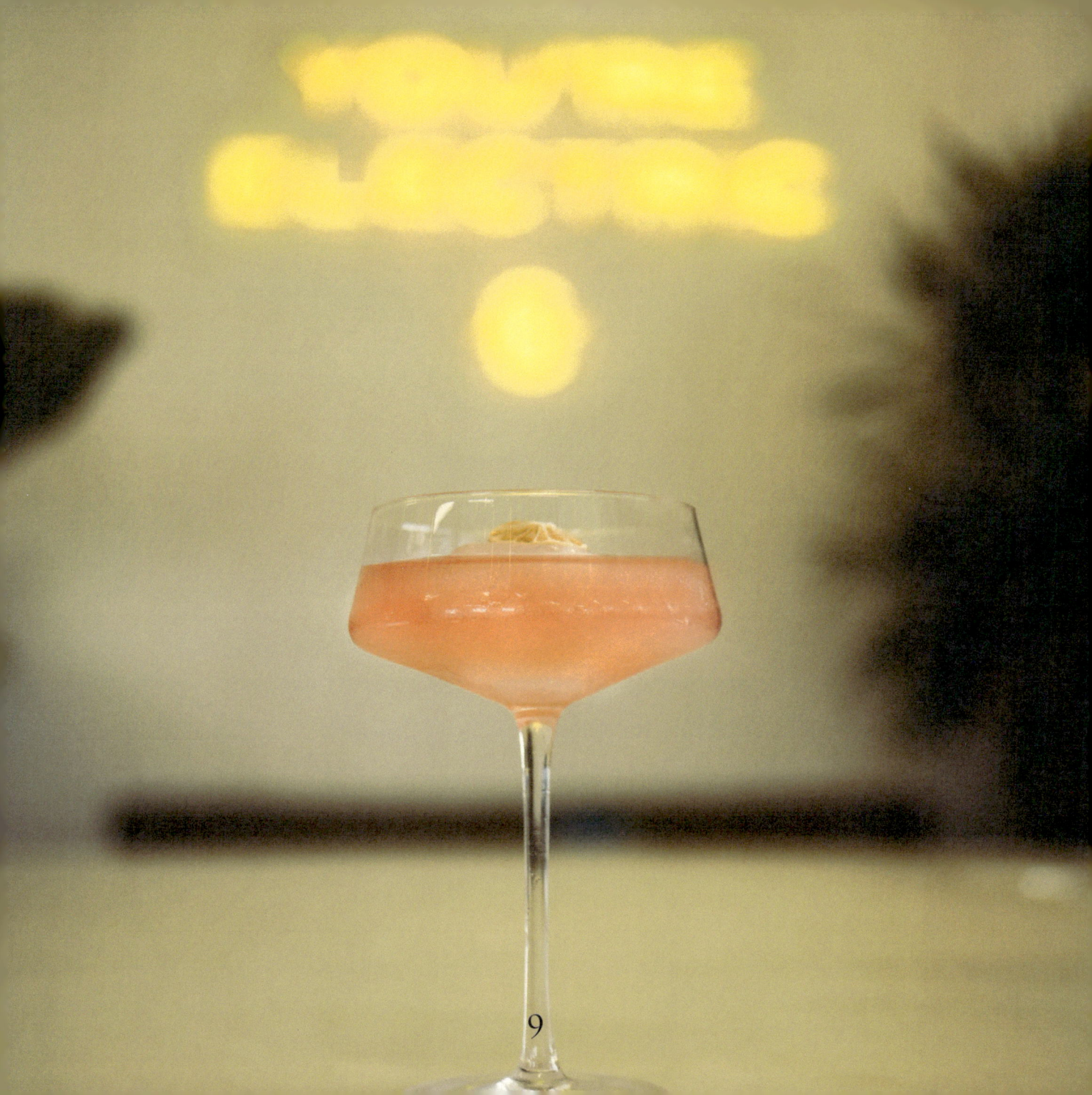

RHUBARB SELTZER
Griffin Brewing Co

Griffin Brewing is a 2 bbl nano brewery located in Enumclaw, WA offering a wide variety of craft beer styles ranging from the lightest lagers to the darkest stouts and everything in between. With 12 house-made beers on tap you're sure to find something you'll enjoy at Griffin Brewing.

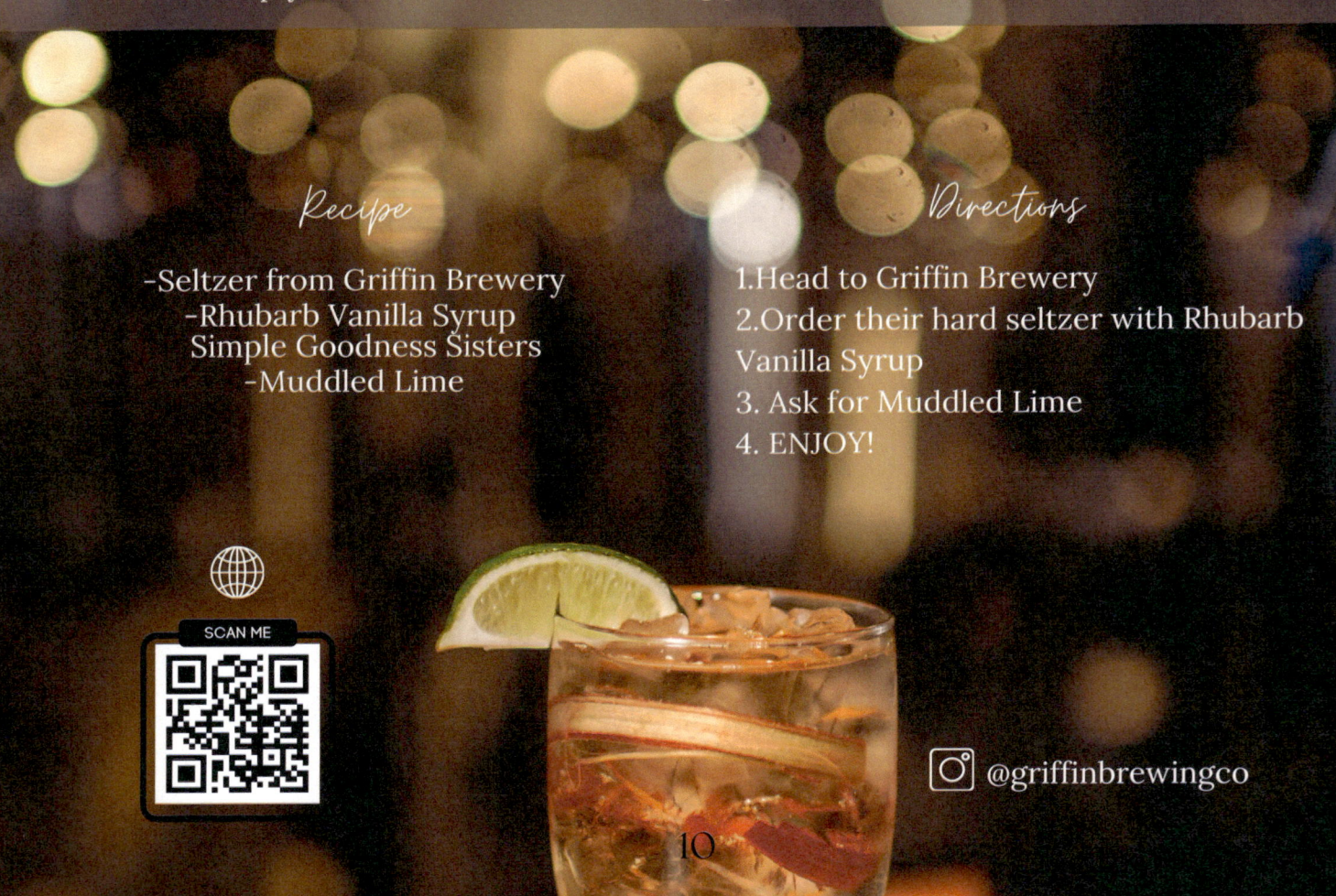

Recipe

- Seltzer from Griffin Brewery
- Rhubarb Vanilla Syrup Simple Goodness Sisters
- Muddled Lime

Directions

1. Head to Griffin Brewery
2. Order their hard seltzer with Rhubarb Vanilla Syrup
3. Ask for Muddled Lime
4. ENJOY!

@griffinbrewingco

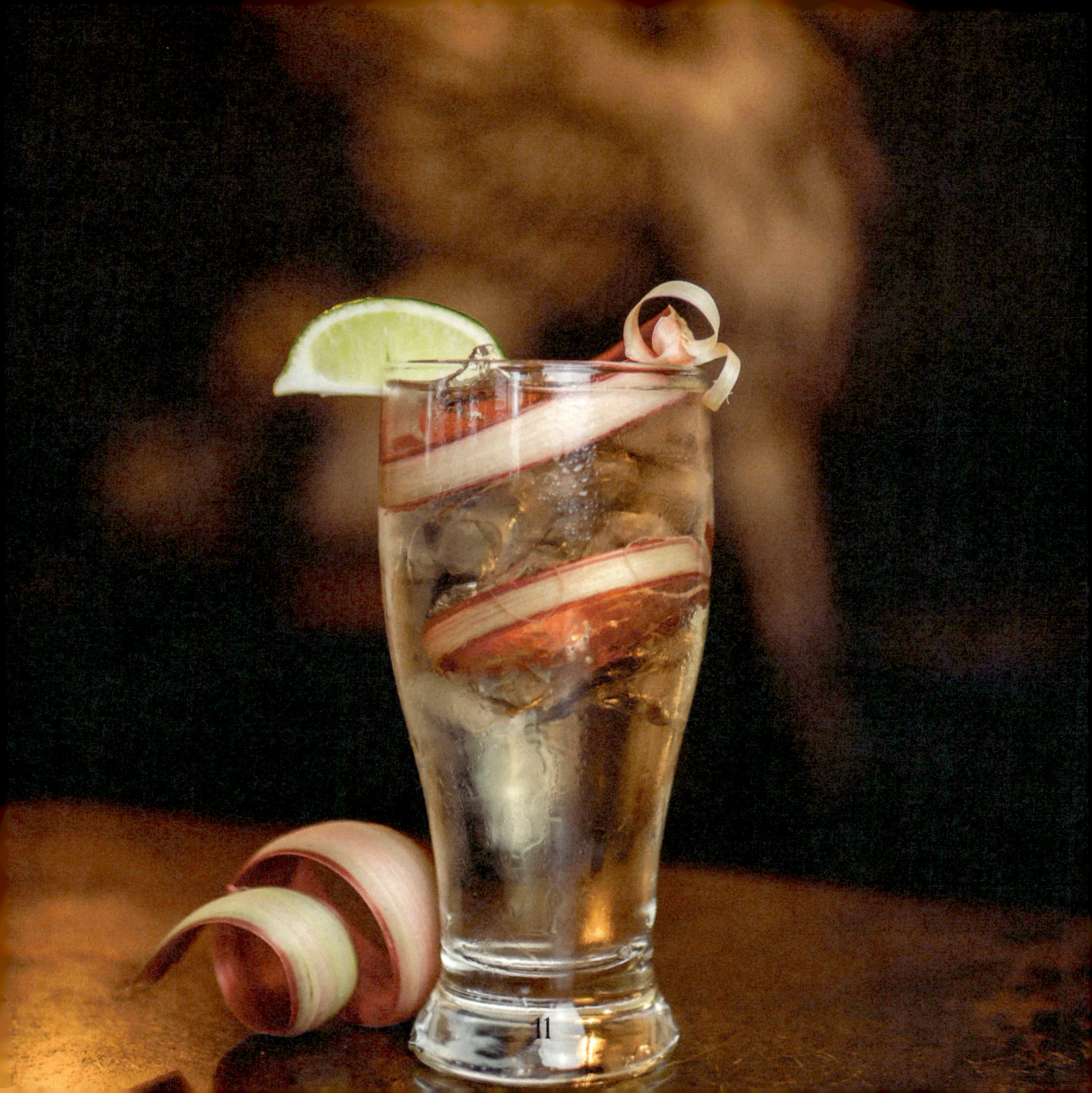

RASPBERRIES & CREAM MARGARITA

Main Street Bistro

Recipe

5-6 Raspberries
1 oz Triple Sec
1 oz Lime Juice
3 oz Tequila
Splash of Raspberry Simple Syrup
1 oz Coconut Cream

Directions

1. Run a lime wedge over the rim of your lowball glass and then dip in salt (or sugar) to coat the rim.
2. Fill the glass with ice and set aside.
3. Add raspberries and Triple Sec to a mixing glass and muddle.
4. Add lime juice, raspberry syrup, Tequila and coconut cream followed by a scoop of ice to the mixing glass.
5. Shake until cold and strain into your cocktail glass.
6. Garnish with a lime wedge and a raspberry or two

@mainstreetbistrobuckley

Main Street Bistro is a family-owned and family-friendly bar and restaurant in Historical Downtown Buckley. In addition to food, beer, wine & spirits, MSB has a full espresso bar, pool and table games and a great selection of handmade gifts to shop from! We are open 7 days aweek, Monday-Friday at 11:30am for lunch and dinner as well as weekend breakfast starting at 9am Saturday & Sunday!

13

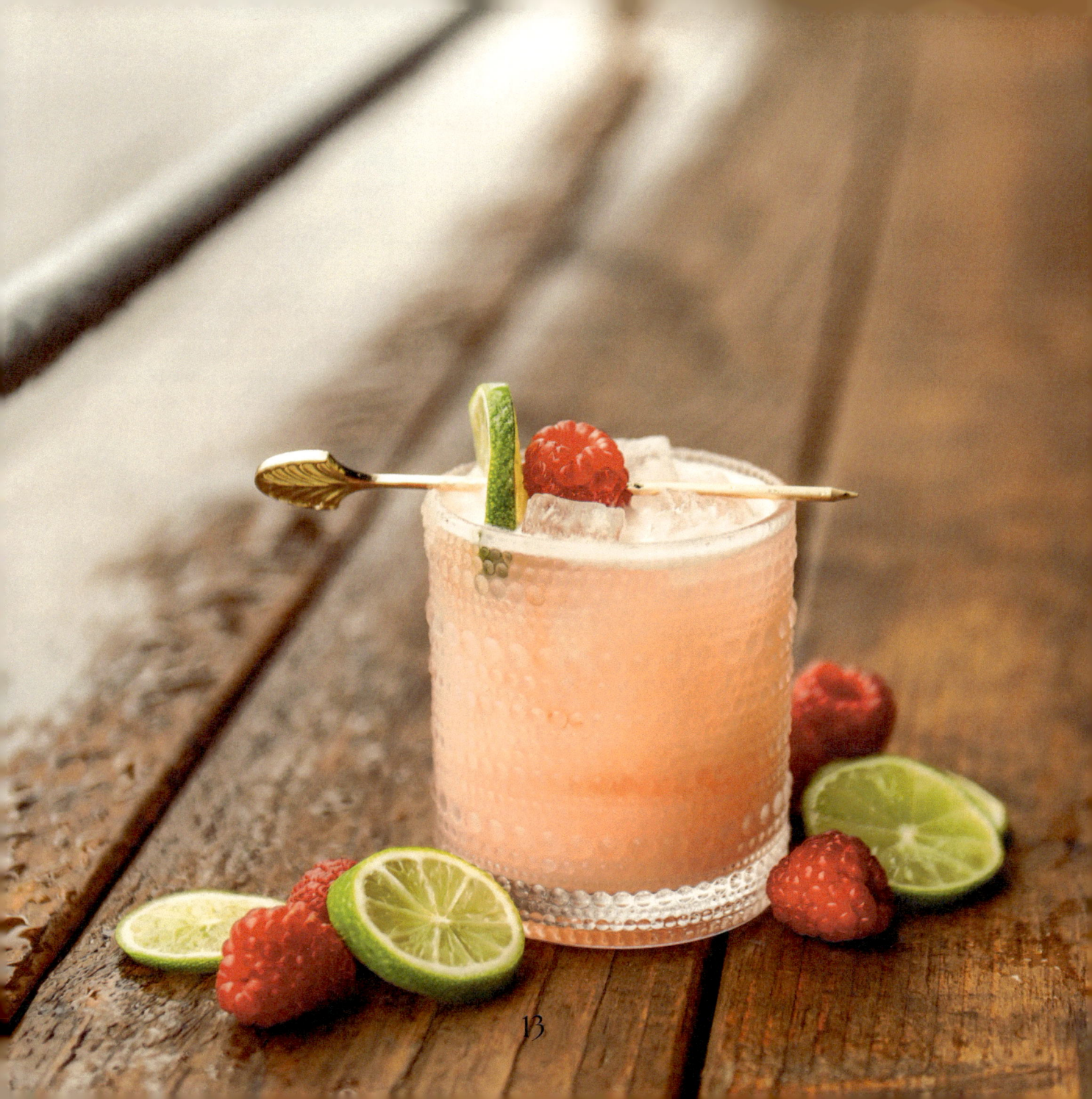

THE GENEVIEVE COCKTAIL
Simple Goodness Sisters

Farmed and handcrafted in the Pacific Northwest, Simple Goodness Sisters syrups capture the intense, pure flavors of a season, and naturally preserve them. We grow the majority of the ingredients for the syrups on our family farm in Buckley, WA and source whatever we can't grow with intention, supporting local farms. The rhubarb for our vanilla rhubarb syrup comes from our own farm as well as our friend's down the valley, Knutson Farms.

With the greatest respect to the ingredients we toil over, the syrups are bottled at our production kitchen at the Simple Goodness Soda Shop, where an infusion of whole fruits, herbs, and spices is added to organic cane sugar and water. Infused with exact timing for maximum flavor, the syrups are deeply flavorful and nuanced, showcasing the unique subtleties of all ingredients. Use them in your drinks at home including cocktails, non-alcoholic drinks, coffee, tea, and sodas. We use only whole fruit, spices and herbs; never any dyes, concentrates, or extracts for our products. Our respect for our time-honored craft is evident in each bottle of pure and delicious syrup

Recipe

Glass: champagne glass or coupe
2 oz Gin
1/2 oz fresh lemon juice
1/2 oz Simple Goodness Sisters Vanilla Rhubarb Syrup
1 ounce brut sparkling wine
Garnish: thin slice rhubarb

Directions

1. Combine the gin, lemon juice and syrup in a shaker of ice
2. Shake for 20 seconds or until the outside of the shaker is chilled.
3. Strain into a coupe glass and top with the sparkling wine.
4. Garnish. Sometimes we use a lemon wheel, sometimes a thin slice of rhubarb that's been dipped in our floral sugar.

@simplegoodnesssisters

15

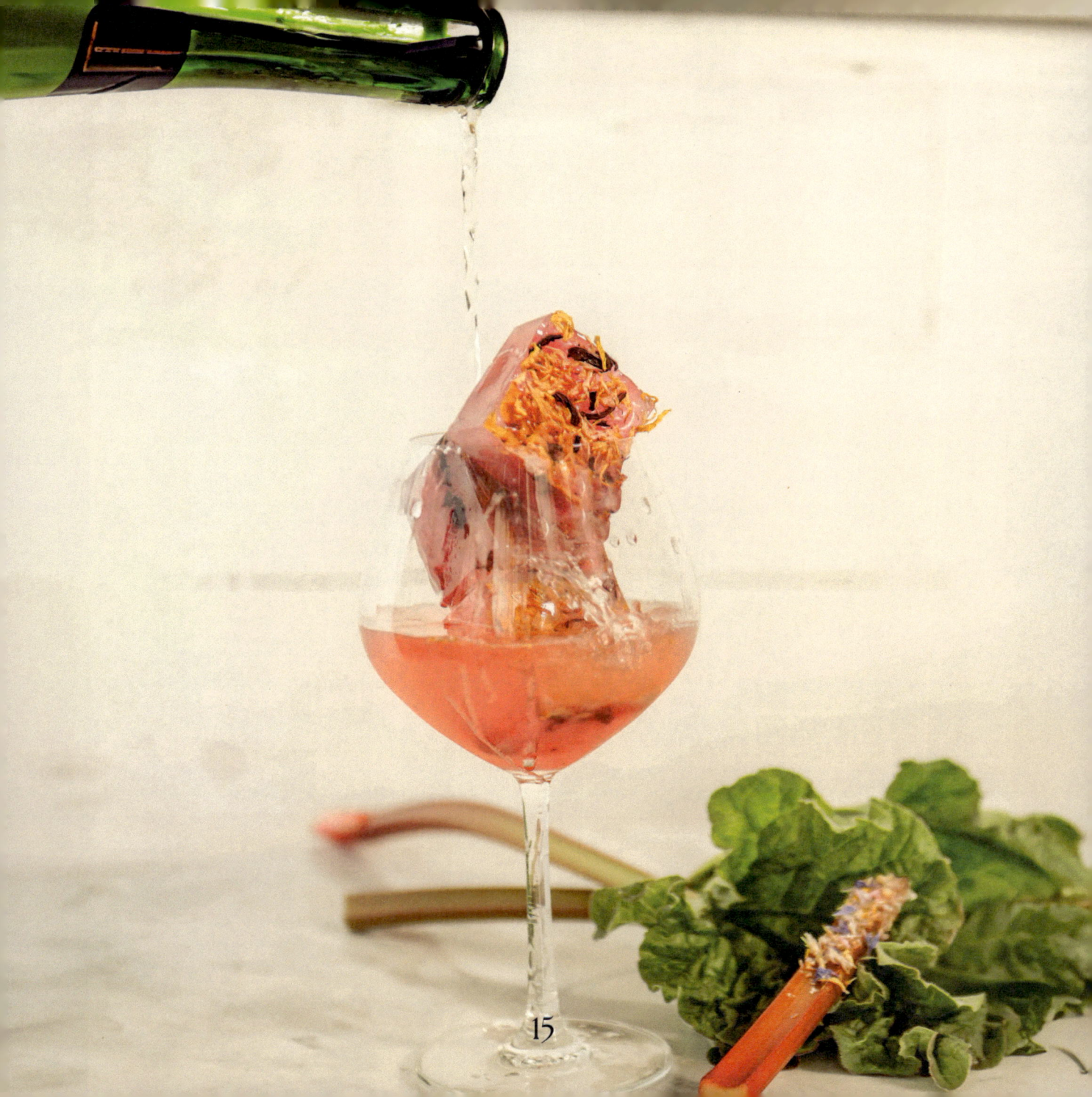

LIMONCELLO MARTINI
Sorci's Italian Café

As a family business, we love traditions - and that's why we had to go with our signature limoncello martini for our selection! Known for our house-made limoncello mix, we use our house infused ingredients with classic flavors to bring an Italian favorite that you can enjoy all year long. We hope you think of us the next time you make this family favorite!

Recipe

2oz vodka
1.5oz limoncello
1.5oz fresh lemon juice
1.5oz simple syrup

Directions

1. Start by adding a sugar rim to your martini glass
2. Add a scoop of ice and pour in the listed ingredients
3. Shake until chilled
4. Strain and pour into a martini glass with sugar rim

Optional: Add 1 oz of raspberry or strawberry purée to do other flavors!

@sorcisitaliancafe

17

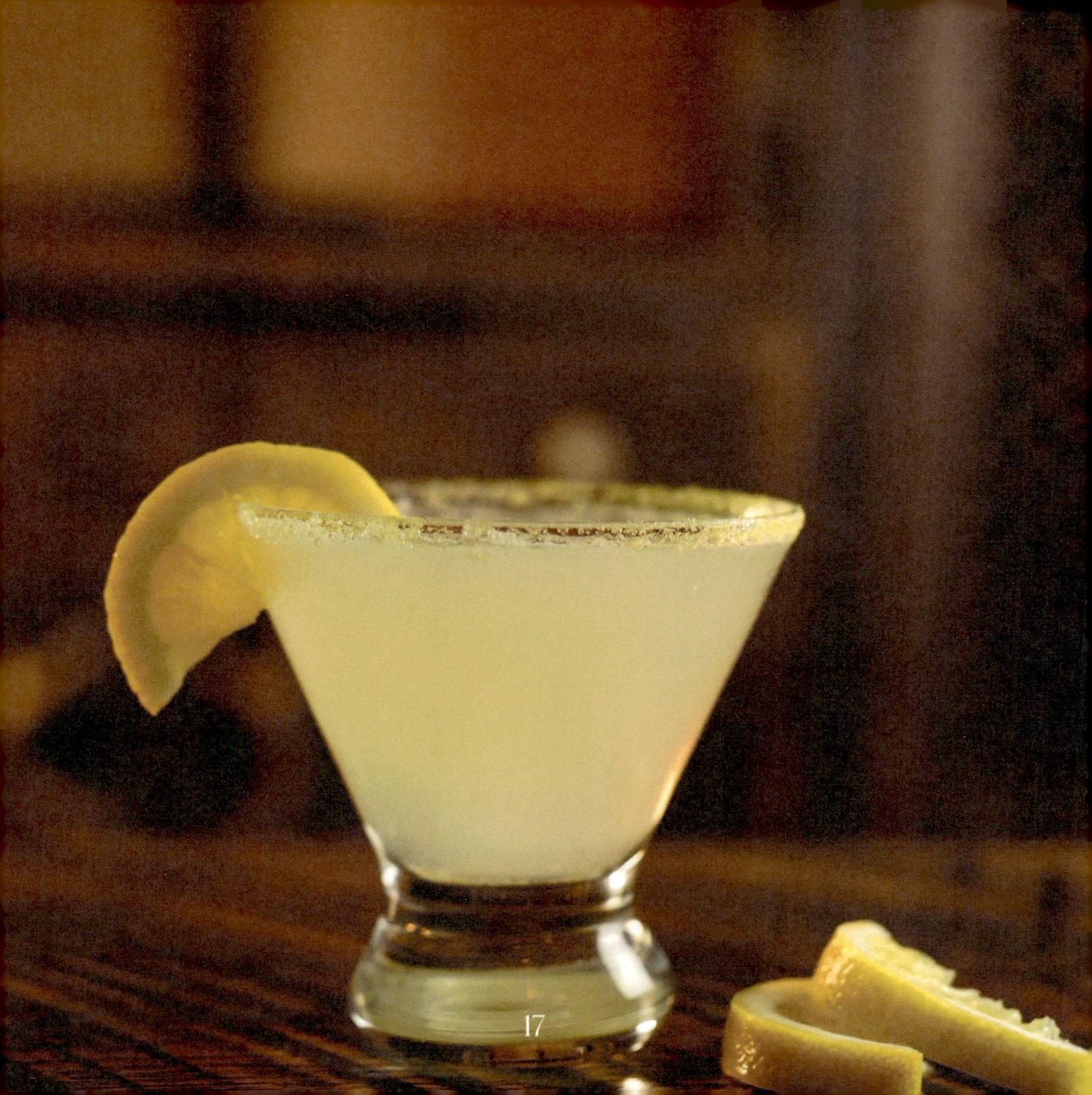

BERRY COBBLER
The Bistro at Windmill Gardens

The Bistro at Windmill Gardens is a family-owned business owned and operated by Chef Bruce Patterson and his wife, Barb Patterson. Our desire is to offer a relaxed, reasonably priced dining experience and focus on creating a memorable guest experience. Already known for exceptional hospitality and high quality service, owner Chef Bruce Patterson has created a menu with a variety of selections sure to please everyone. With a motto of Grand Simplicity, he lets the ingredients speak for themselves.

The Bistro at Windmill Gardens offers lunch, happy hour and dinner as well as offering breakfast on weekends. We invite you to be our guest and hope your first visit will be one of many!

Recipe

- 3 raspberries
- 2 blackberries
- 2 oz Tito's Vodka
- 3/4 oz Cocchi American Aperitif
- 1/2 oz Simple Syrup
- 3/4 oz Lemon Juice

Directions

1. Muddle the raspberries and blackberries in pint glass
2. Add ice, Tito's Vodka, Cocchi, simple syrup, and lemon juice
3. Cover with shaker and shake vigorously
4. Double strain into a Coupe glass.
5. Garnish with skewer with one of each berry.

Cheers!

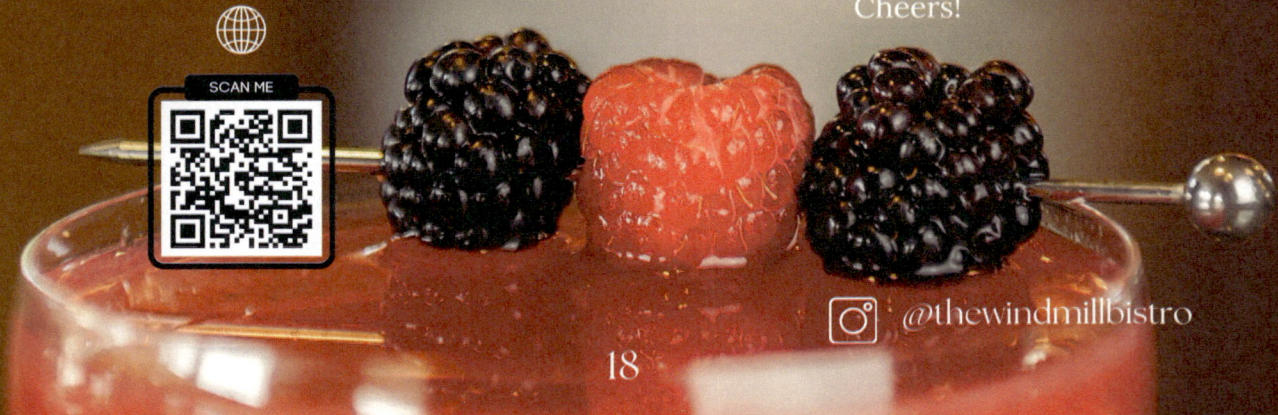

@thewindmillbistro

19

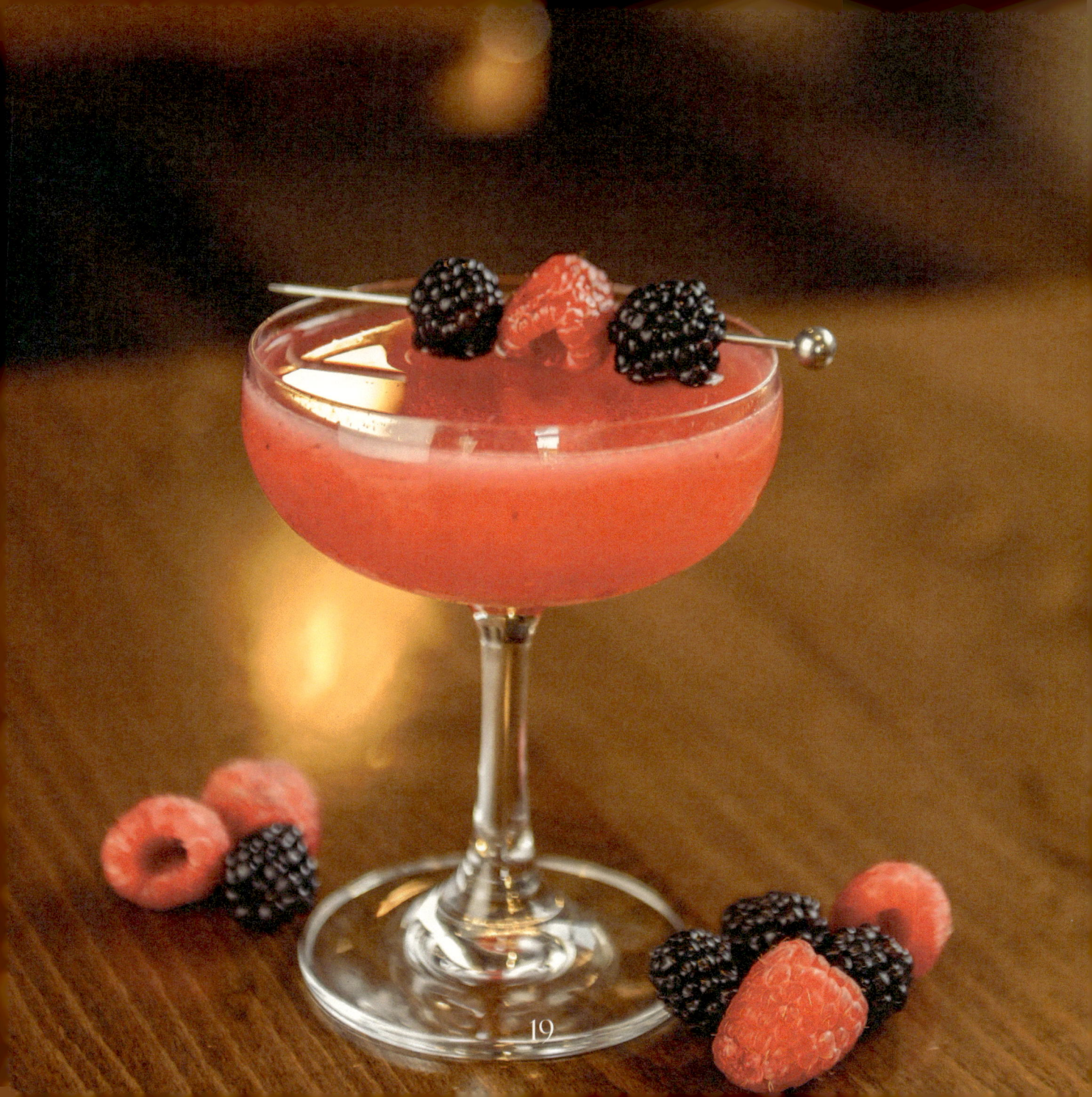

HOT PARADISE
The Bistro at Windmill Gardens

Recipe

2 oz El Jimador Tequila
½ oz lemon juice
¾ oz Caribbean Pineapple Liqueur
¾ oz spicy Agave Syrup
1 oz Pineapple Juice
3 dashes Angosturra bitters

Directions

1. Add all ingredients to a shaker tin with ice.
2. Cover with pounder glass and shake vigorously.
3. Strain into rocks glass and add fresh ice.

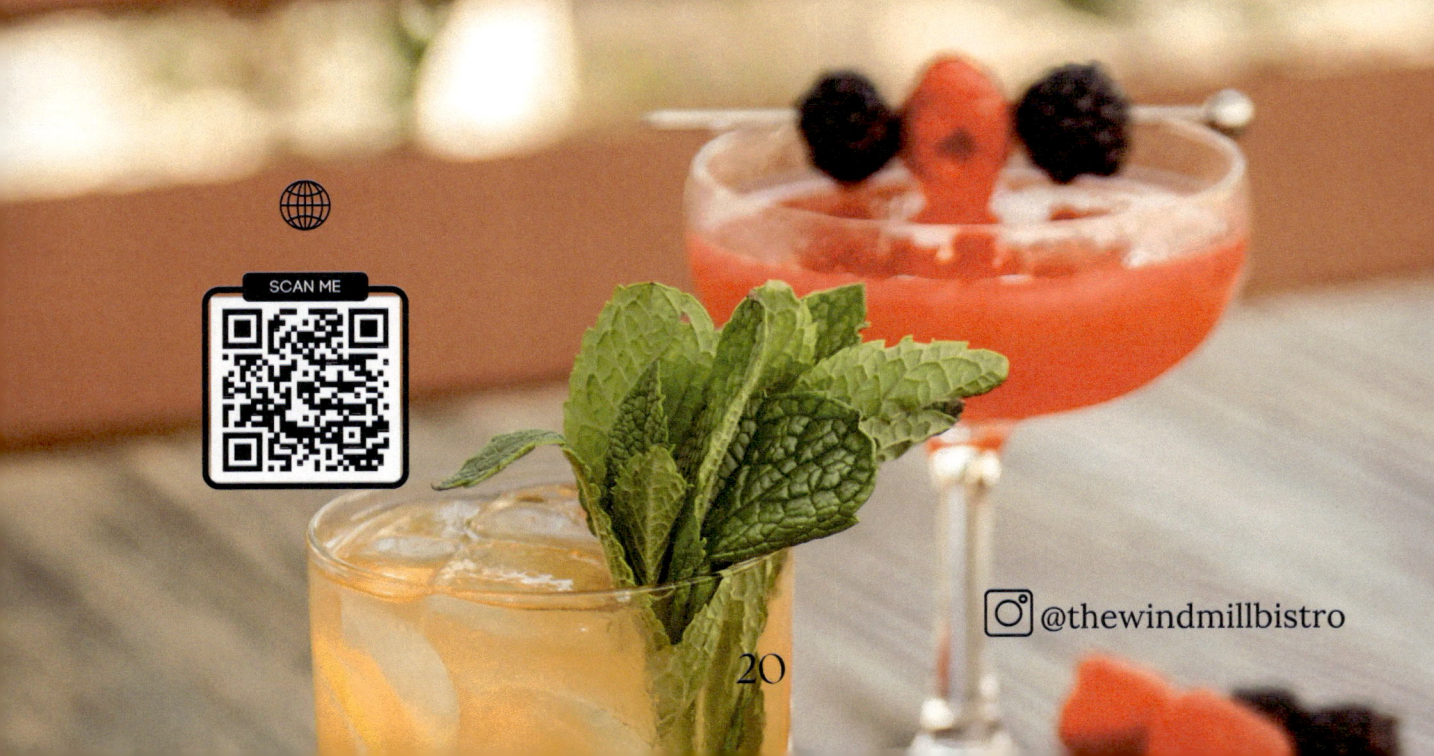

@thewindmillbistro

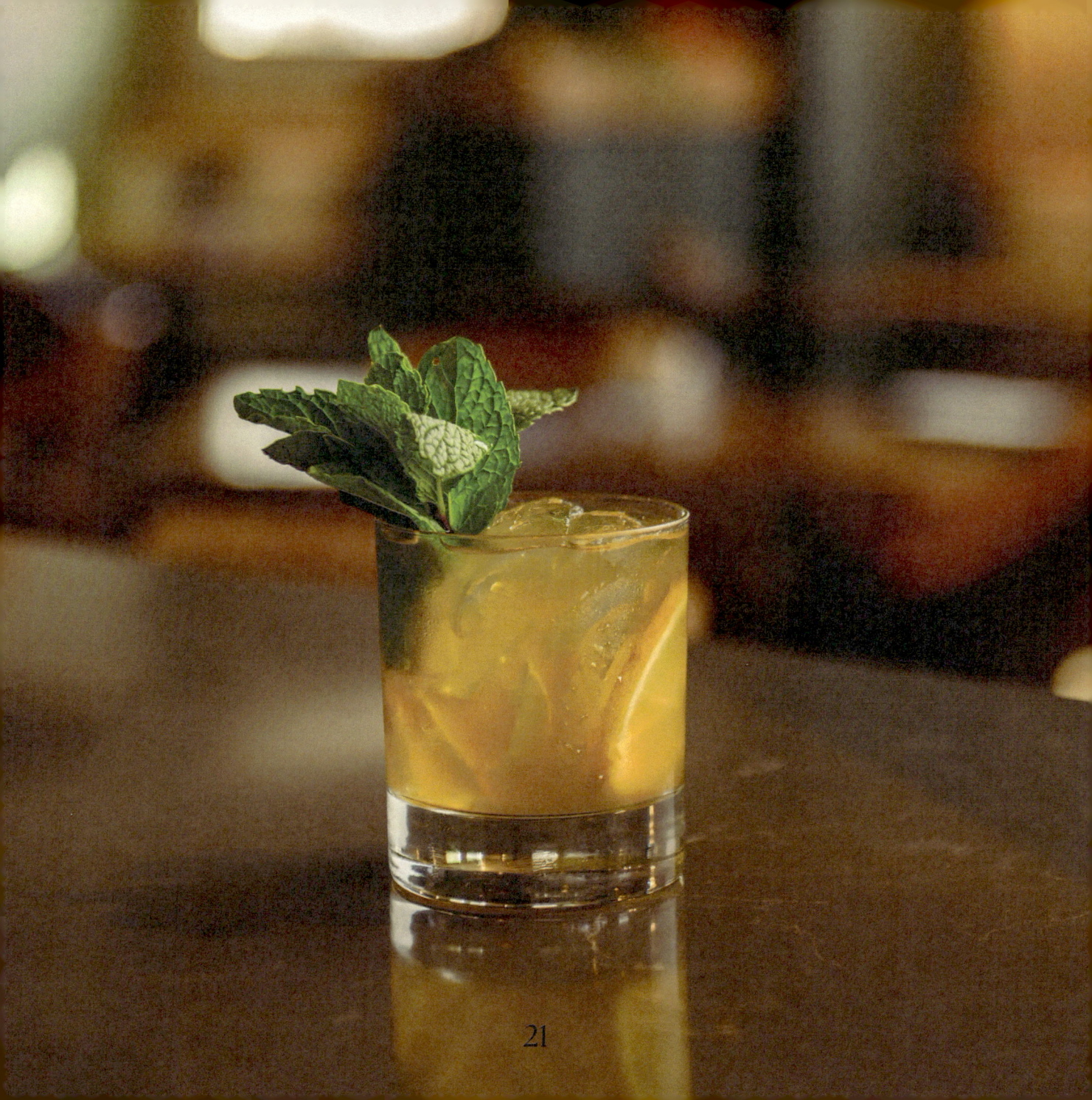

FIERCE COUNTY GINGER RYE
Fierce County Cider

Recipe

6 oz Fierce County Cider's Gin Gin Cran
1 oz Heritage Dual Barrel Rye Whiskey
1/2oz simple syrup
Orange garnish

Directions

1. Add ice to a glass
2. Add in cider, simple syrup and whiskey
3. Stir to combine ingredients
4. Garnish with an orange twist Enjoy!

@fiercecounty

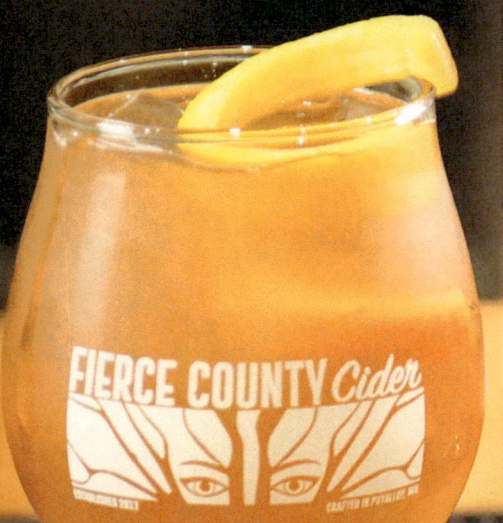

23

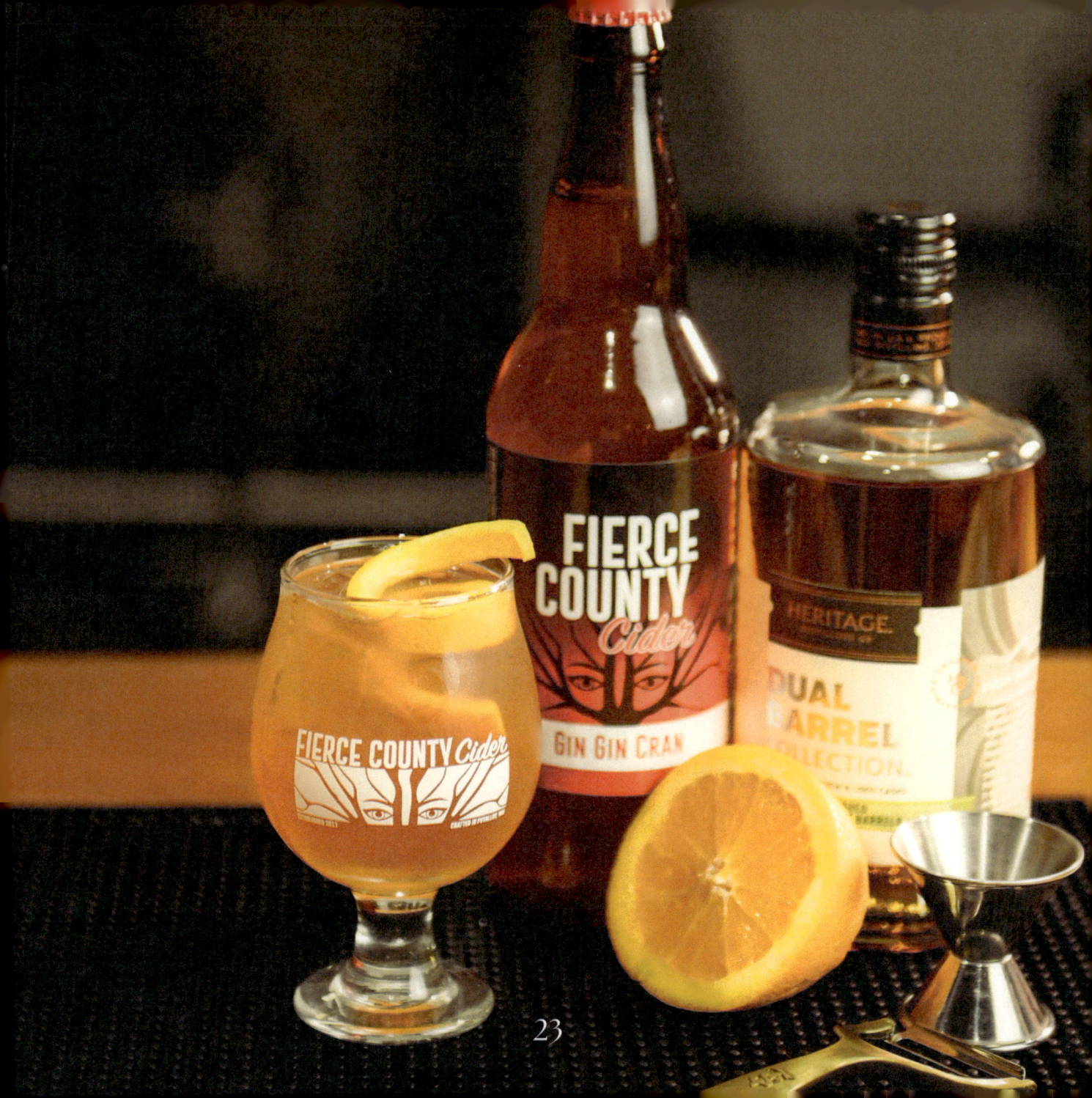

INTA PINK
Inta Vintage

Dive into our marketplace wonderland! We're a treasure trove of goodies with 60 vendors and 3 floors. From timeless antiques to funky vintage vibes, and handmade wonders to repurposed gems– we've got it all!

Recipe

1 oz coconut rum
1 oz light rum
1 oz pineapple juice
1 oz lemonade
1.5 oz blueberry lemonade

Directions

1. Mix all ingredients together with ice in a shaker
2. Pour into your favorite vintage cocktail glass from Inta Vintage
3. Serve with a slice of fresh pineapple.
4. Enjoy!

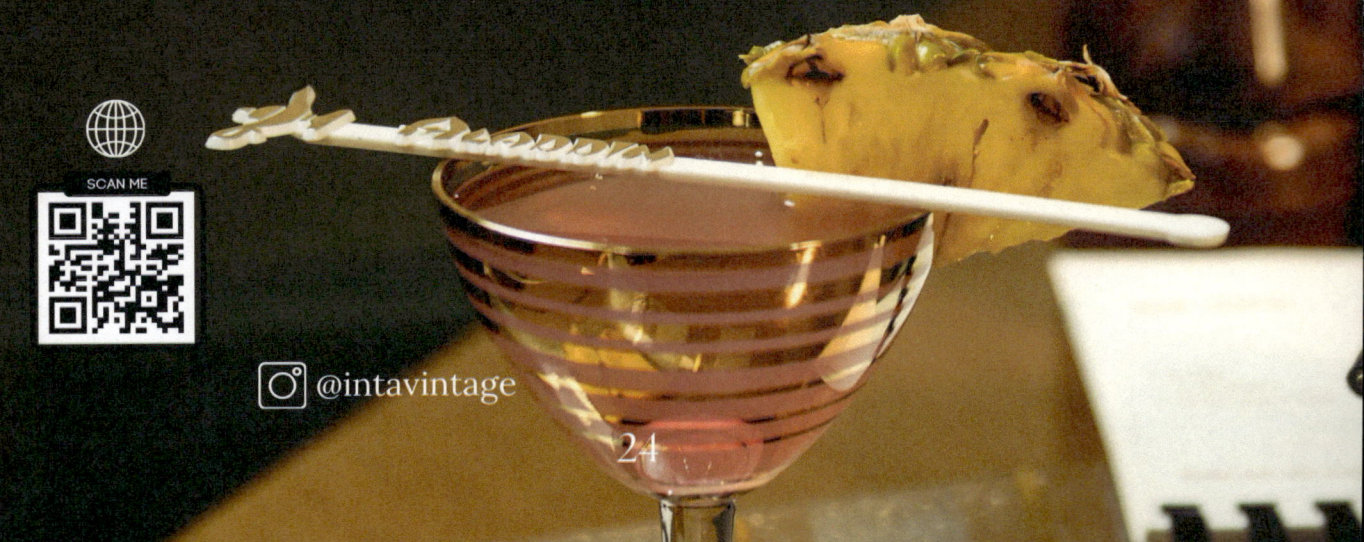

Barware: @vintagekupkake
Setting: @macs_vintage_market

@intavintage

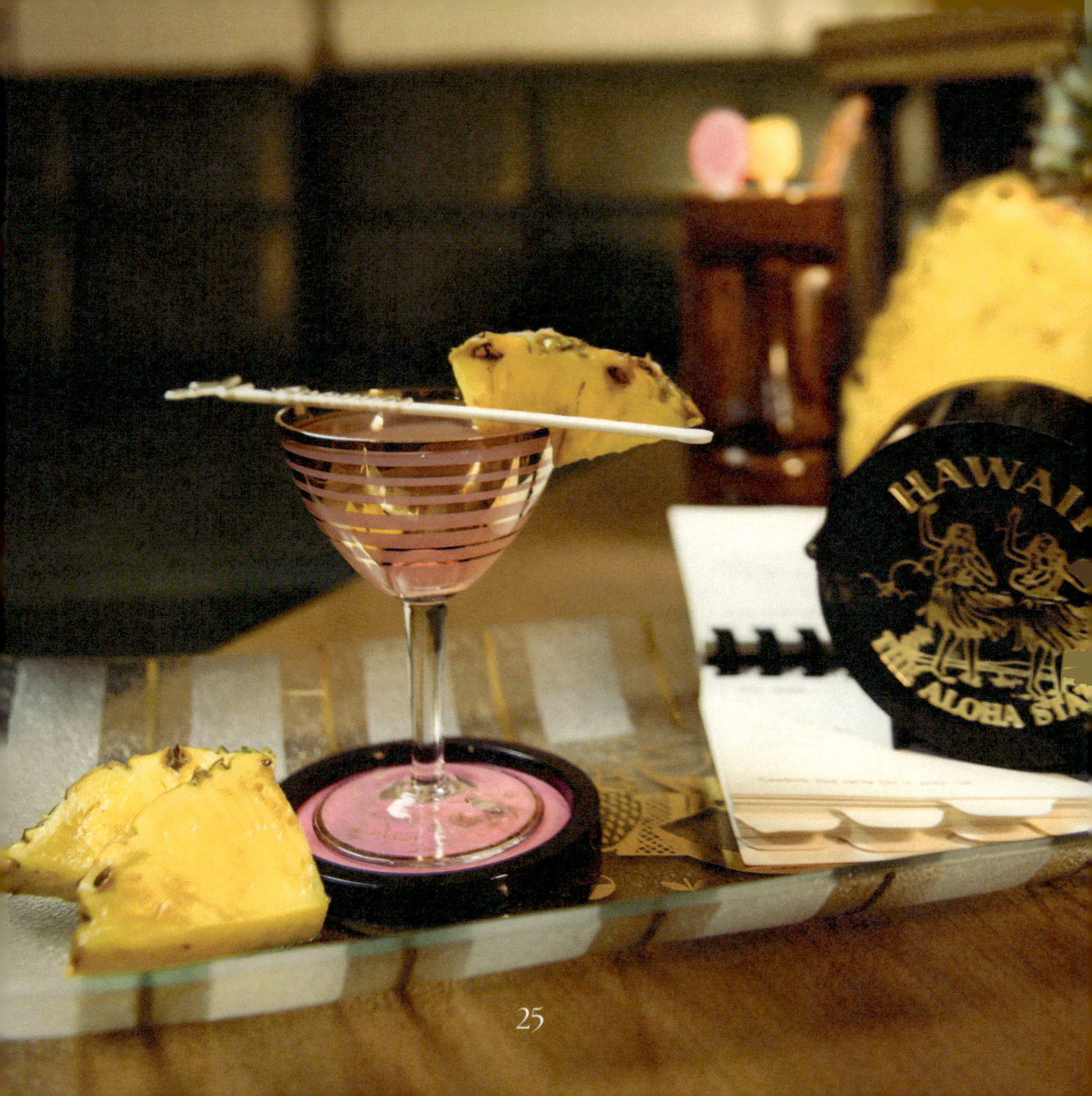

STRAWBERRY RHUBARB LEMONADE
Knutson Farms Inc

Fresh Pressed Lemonade

1 juicy lemon
1/3 cup sugar
2 cups water
1 cup ice

Shake all Ingredients vigorously.

Strawberry Rhubarb Simple Syrup

2.5 cups rhubarb, chopped
1/2 cup strawberries, chopped
1 cup sugar
1 cup water

Bring all ingredients to a boil. Simmer for 20 minutes. Strain with fine strainer or cheese cloth. This recipe makes 1 cup simple syrup.

Use 1 oz. simple syrup for each glass of fresh pressed lemonade!

@knutsonfarmsinc

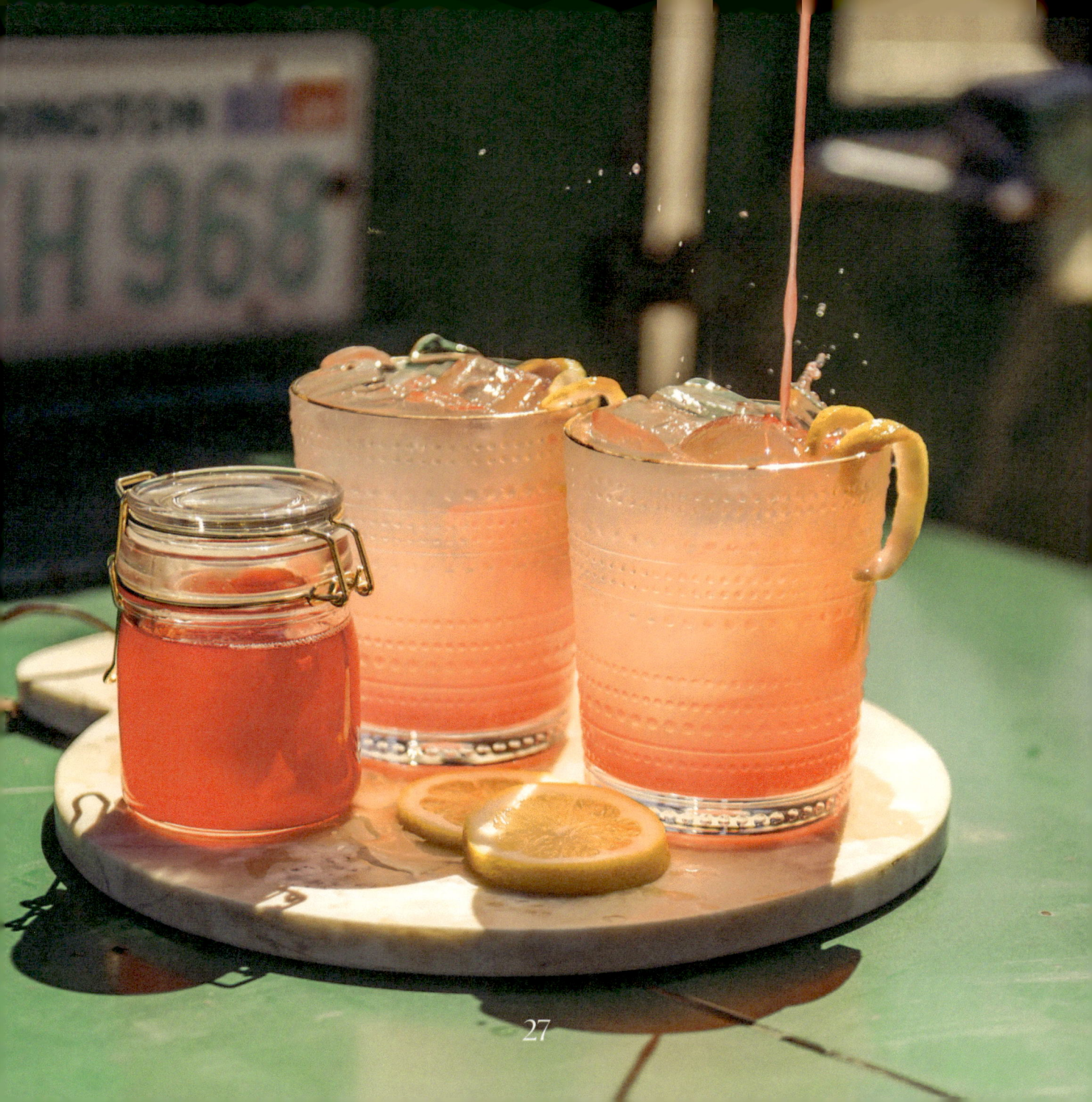

GINGER MARGARTIA
Locale Plants

Recipe

2 oz tequila
1/2 oz orange liquer
1 oz fresh lime juice
Ginger beer
Kosher salt for rim
Fresh lime for garnish

Directions

1. Use a lime wedge to wet rim of glass and roll rim in kosher salt
2. Stir tequila, orange liqueur and lime juice together.
3. Add crushed ice. Top off with ginger beer.
4. Add a circle of lime if you're fancy.

www.localeplants.com

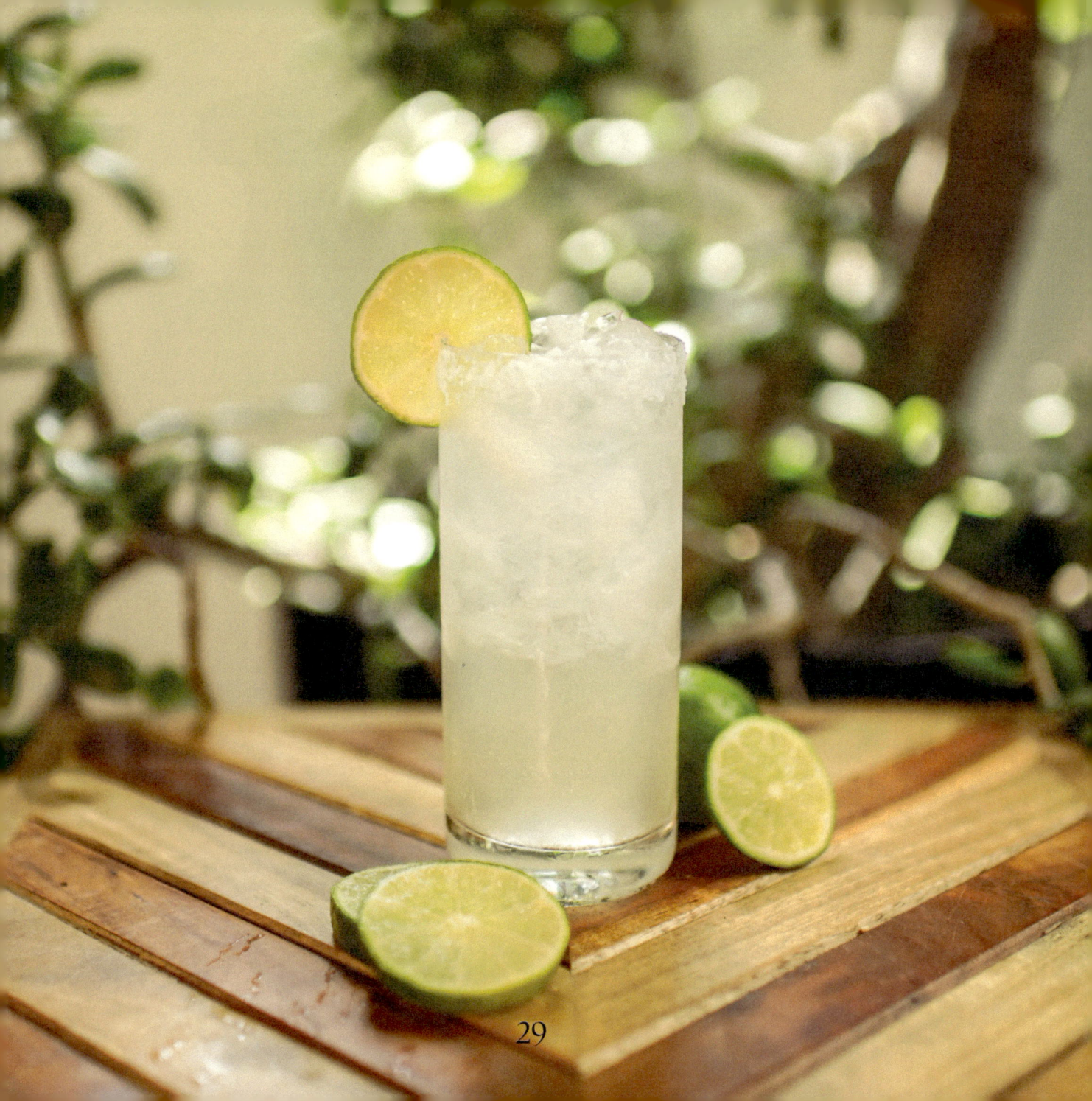

DIRTY MARTINI
Bomb Charcuterie

We are a small, locally-owned business that has been serving the community for three years. Excitingly, we will be opening our first physical location in Sumner this summer! Specializing in artisanal cheese, charcuterie, sandwiches, and tartines, we are dedicated to providing high-quality, delicious food options. Additionally, we will be offering workshops, provisions, and a variety of unique gifts. We are thrilled to embark on this new chapter and look forward to becoming a staple in the Sumner-Puyallup community.

Recipe

3 oz Belvedere vodka
2.5 oz Mezzetta Colossal Castelvetrano Brine + 3 olives
Splash of Dolin Vermouth
Artisanal Blue Cheese

Directions

1. Place martini glass in the freezer.
2. In a small bowl mix blue cheese and a splash of vodka
3. Pipe into olives.
4. Rinse glass with vermouth, discard the excess and place back into the freezer.
3. In a cocktail shaker full of ice, pour in vodka and olive brine
4. Shake the cocktail shaker 50 times and pour into the martini glass.
Enjoy!

SCAN ME

www.bombcharcuterie.com

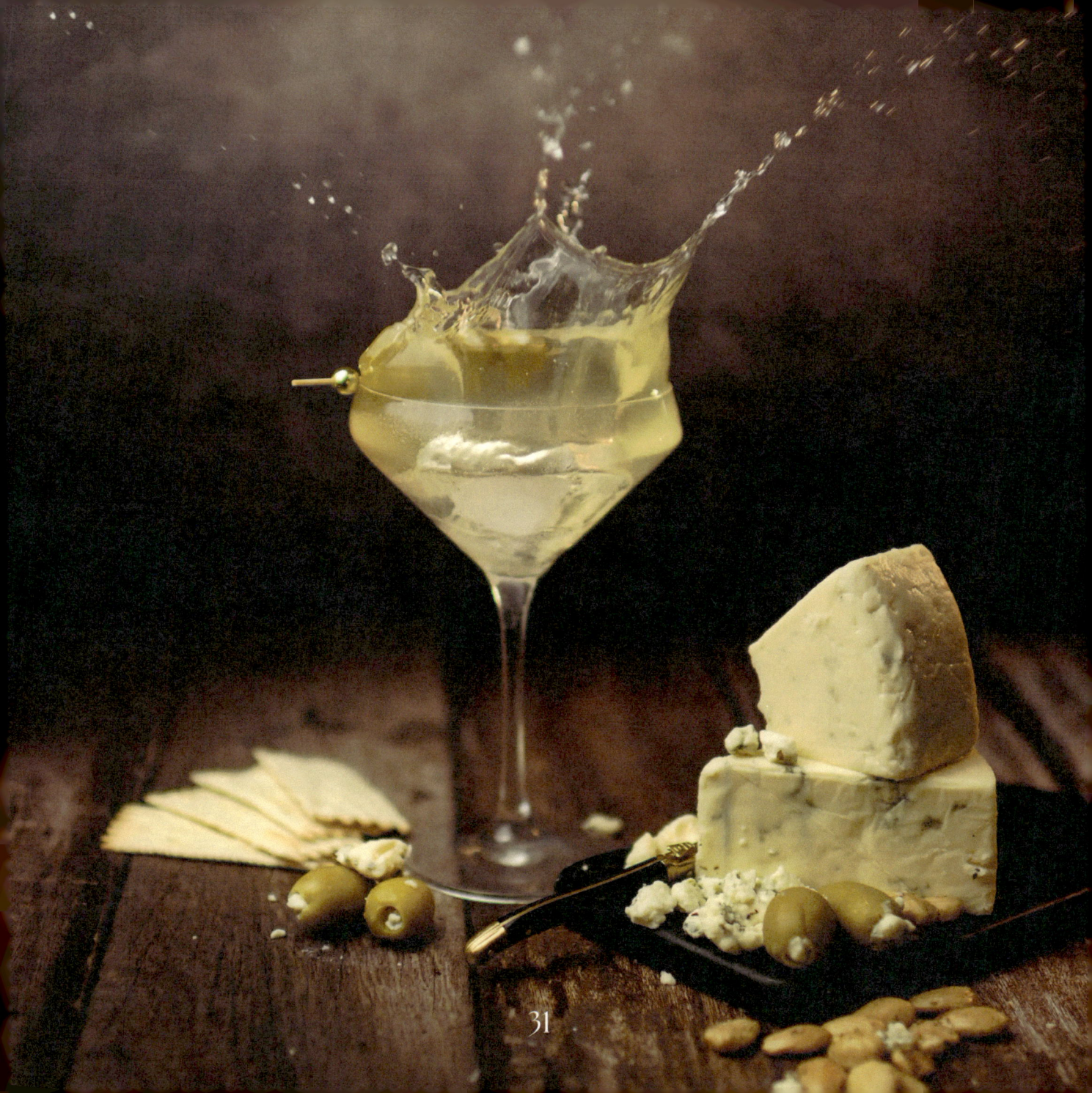

JUNGLE CAT
Township 20

This exotic blend of tropical fruits, herbs, and Whiskey has historic roots in a cocktail called the Jungle Bird. If you like it, try it with Rum next time! And if you are a coffee fan, add a dash of cold brew to your cocktail for the Midnight Jungle experience.

Recipe

1.5oz Jack Daniel's Tennessee Whiskey
2oz pineapple juice
1/2oz Carpano Bitter (Or Campari)
3/4oz lime juice
1/2oz simple syrup (Dissolve sugar into water in equal parts, a 1:1 ratio)
Dash salt

Directions

1. Shake everything together in a cocktail shaker with plenty of ice for about 12 seconds.
2. Pour the mixture over ice
3. Add a couple of Pineapple Fronds to the glass to mimic the ears of the Jungle Cat.

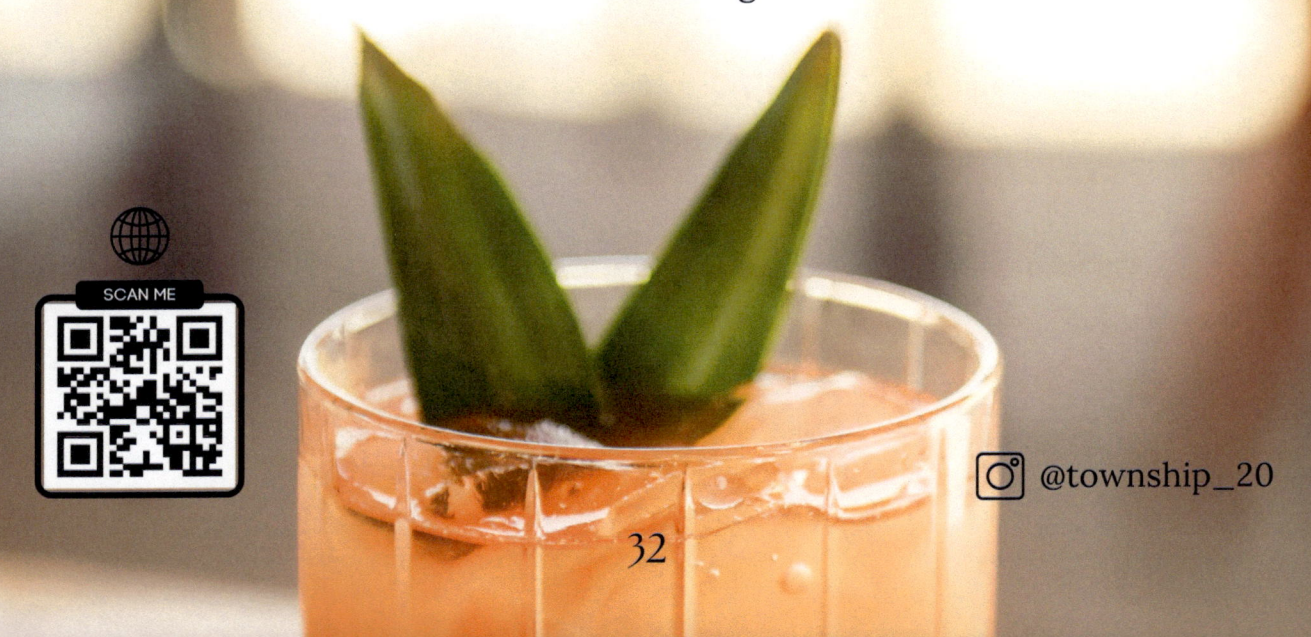

@township_20

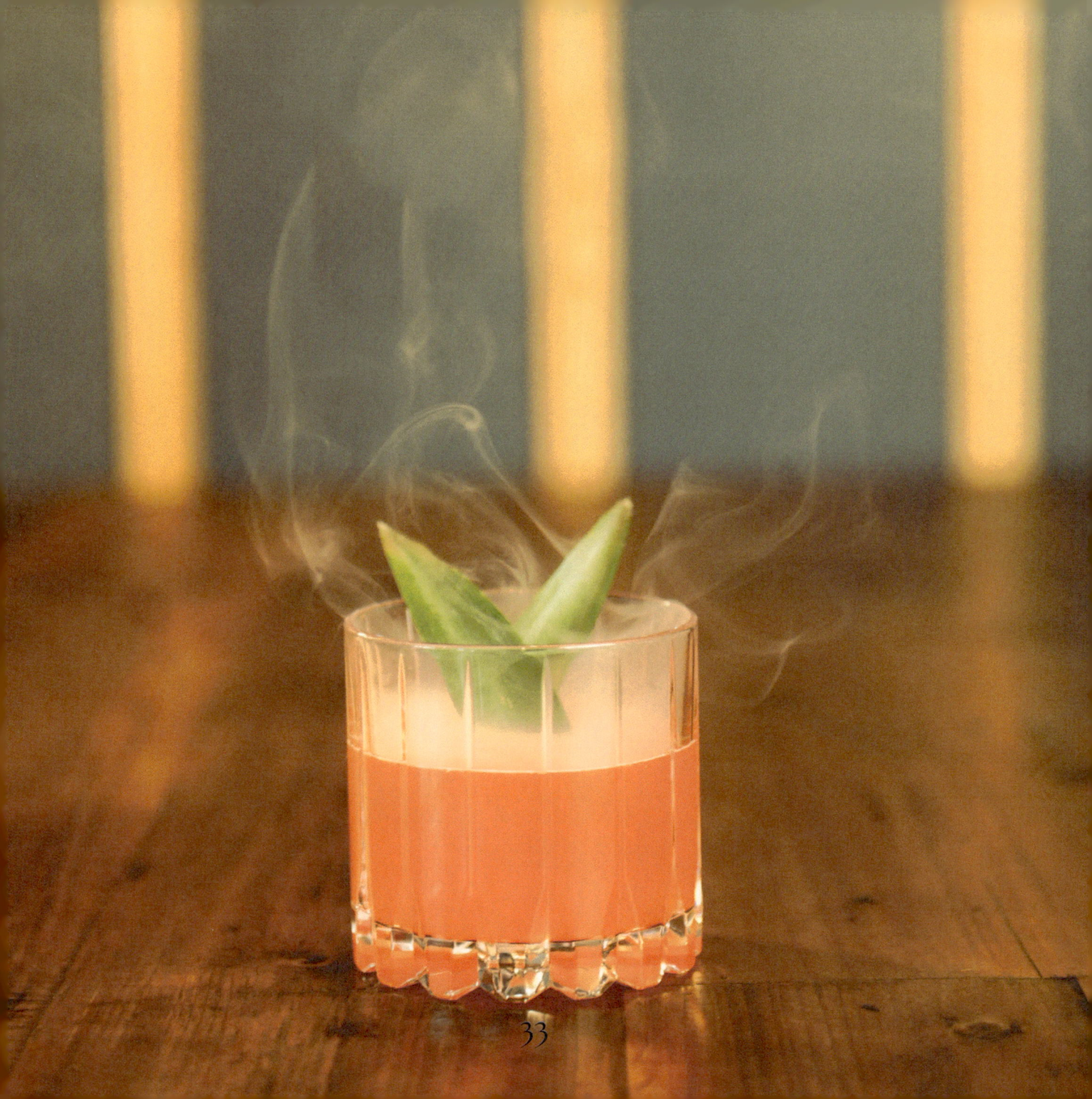

RHAPPLE RHARDAMOM SPRITZ
Township_20

Rhubarb seems to find its way into everything, and we love that about Sumner! So you've had Rhubarb Pie, Rhubarb Crumble, and maybe even Rhubarb Muffins, but have you ever gotten to enjoy a sunny Summer day, sipping on Rhubarb? We Slow-simmer Fresh Rhubarb with Local Apples, Cardamom Pods, and Apple Cider Vinegar to create a Soda Sensation that dates back to the 1600s.

Not only is this recipe delicious, it's also easy to alter into an infinite variety of homemade sodas. Substitute in your favorite Fruits, Herbs, and Vegetables for the Rhubarb, Apple, and Cardamom to create a new and interesting tonic.

Recipe

1.33 cups water, heated
1.33 cups sugar
1/2 cups rhubarb, chopped
1/2 cups apple, chopped
5-8 cardamom pods (to taste)
3/4 cups apple cider vinegar
Pinch of Salt

Directions

1. Dissolve the sugar in hot water on the stove
2. Chop up the apples and rhubarb.
3. Add the apples and rhubarb to the dissolved sugar mixture and bring to a simmer.
4. Simmer for 30 minutes.
5. Add the apple cider vinegar and cardamom pods and simmer for an additional 30 minutes.
6. Strain the mixture, add a dash of salt, and refrigerate.

*This mix should last in the refrigerator for at least two weeks.

@township_20

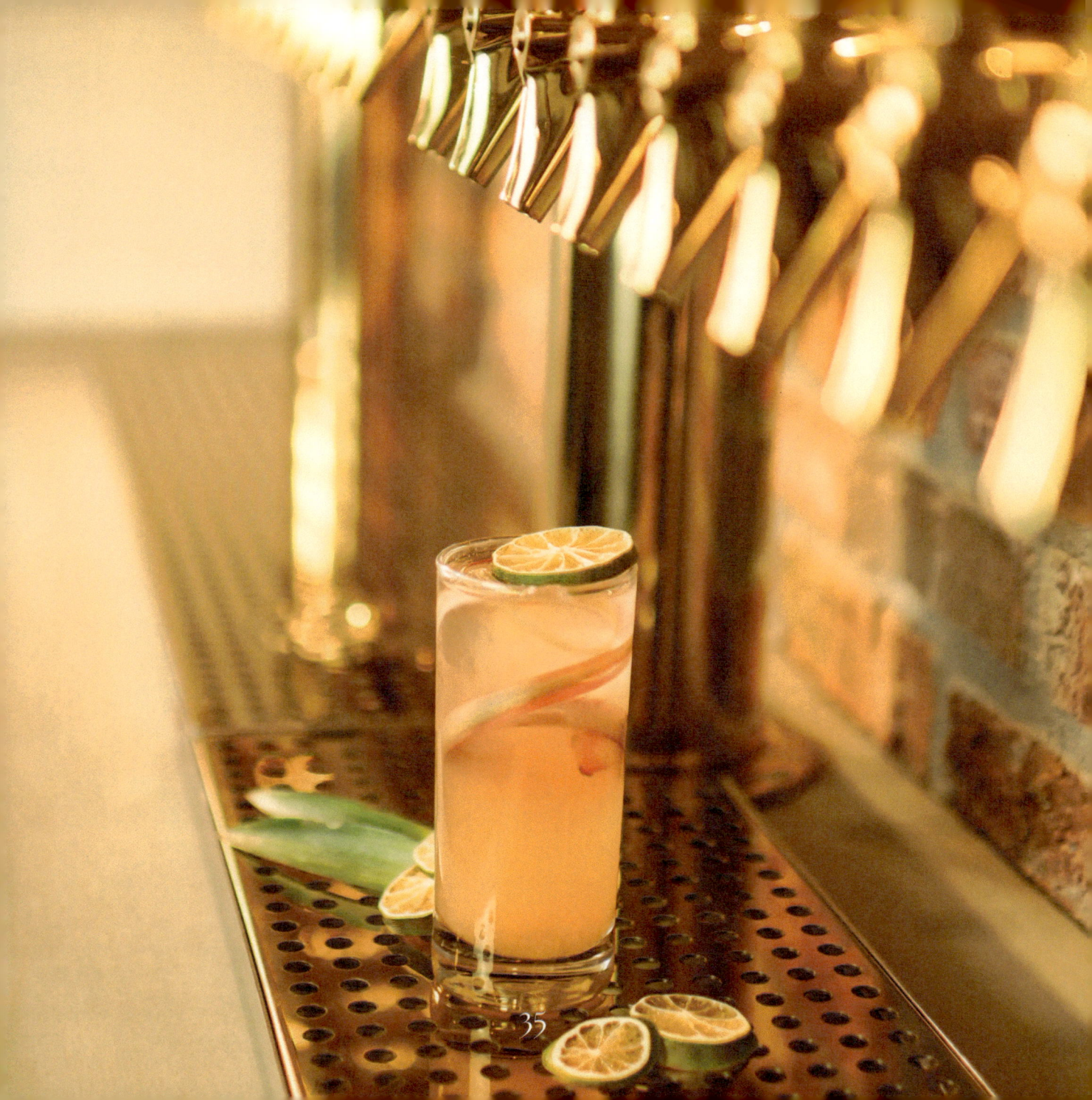

A LITTLE GINGER ON YOUR MIND AMERICANO
Untamed Coffee & Muddy Soda

At Untamed Coffee & Muddy Soda we are here to bring you the best coffee and beverages you have ever had. We don't cut corners on quality. Our goal is to turn you into a coffee snob and know the flavor of an exquisite coffee. As a Woman and Firefighter Owned business we know how hard work and dedication needs to be the heart of everything we do. Don't forget to come try the simple drinks like a cappuccino, a doppio, or one of our Cortado's.

Recipe

12 oz Americano (Can be made hot or iced)
1 Tbs fresh ginger extract (Suja Ginger Shots works great)
1/2 Tbs honey
2 Shots of espresso
Ice
Sparkling water
Hibiscus cold foam

Directions

Add to your cup:
1. Fresh Ginger Extract and Honey
2. Pour espresso over the ginger and honey
3. Add 1/2 cup ice
4. Fill cup to 3/4 full with sparkling water
5. Top it with a hibiscus cold foam

SCAN ME

www.untamedcoffeeco.com

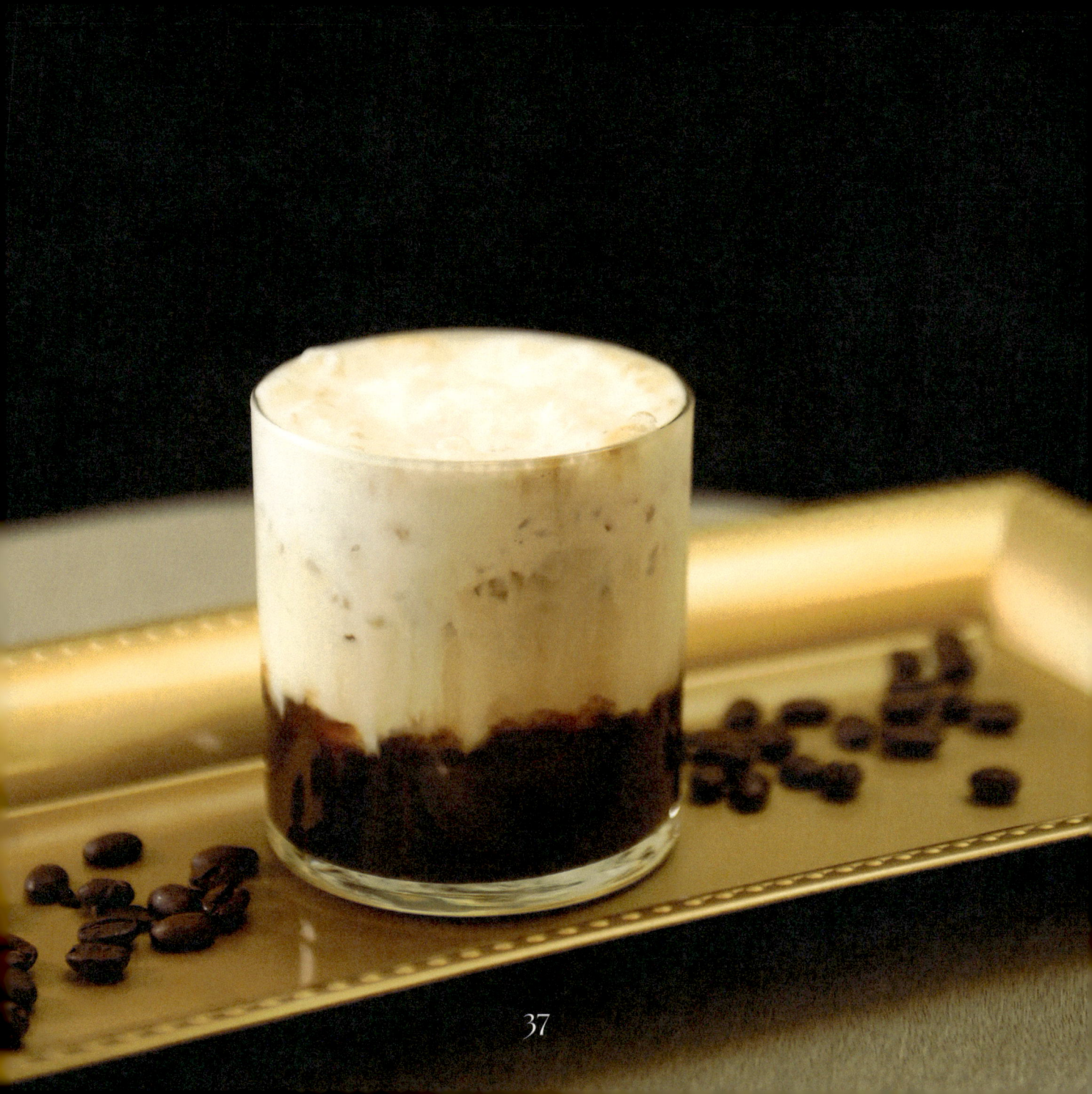

GINGER DROPS
Untamed Coffee & Muddy Soda

Recipe

1.5 Tbs of Fresh Ginger Extract (we use Suva Ginger Shots)
-1 oz of Hibiscus Syrup
Sparkling water
Lemonade
Fresh sliced ginger
Dried Hibiscus flowers

Directions

Grab that 16 oz glass:
1. Add 1.5 Tbs of fresh ginger extract and 1 oz of hibiscus syrup
2. Fill half the glass with ice
3. Fill 2/3 of the glass with sparkling water
4. Top the drink with lemonade
5. Garnish with fresh sliced ginger and some dried hibiscus flowers

www.untamedcoffeeco.com

WHAT THE GINGER MUDDY SODA
Untamed Coffee & Muddy Soda

Recipe

1.5 Ttbs ginger extract
(we use Suja Ginger Shots)
1 oz Hibiscus Syrup
Ginger Ale
Lemonade
Fresh Ginger Slices
Dried Hibiscus flowers

Directions

1. Grab that 16 oz glass
2. Add ginger extract and hibiscus syrup
3. Fill 1/2 the glass with ice
4. Use half ginger ale and half lemonade to fill the glass
5. Give it a good stir
6. Garnish with fresh ginger slices & dried hibiscus flowers

SMOOTHARITA
Eternal Soul Bowl

Recipe

1 cup frozen pineapple
1 cup frozen mango
1 cup banana
1 whole kiwi
1 cup apple juice
1/3 cup lime juice
1 cup frozen Kale/spinach
1 tsp hemp seeds
1 tbs agave
Tahini rim

Directions

1. Rim a tall glass with Tajin
2. Add all ingredients to a blender
3. Blend!
4. Pour smoothie into glass
5. Sprinkle with Tajin
6. Garnish with a lime wedge
Enjoy!

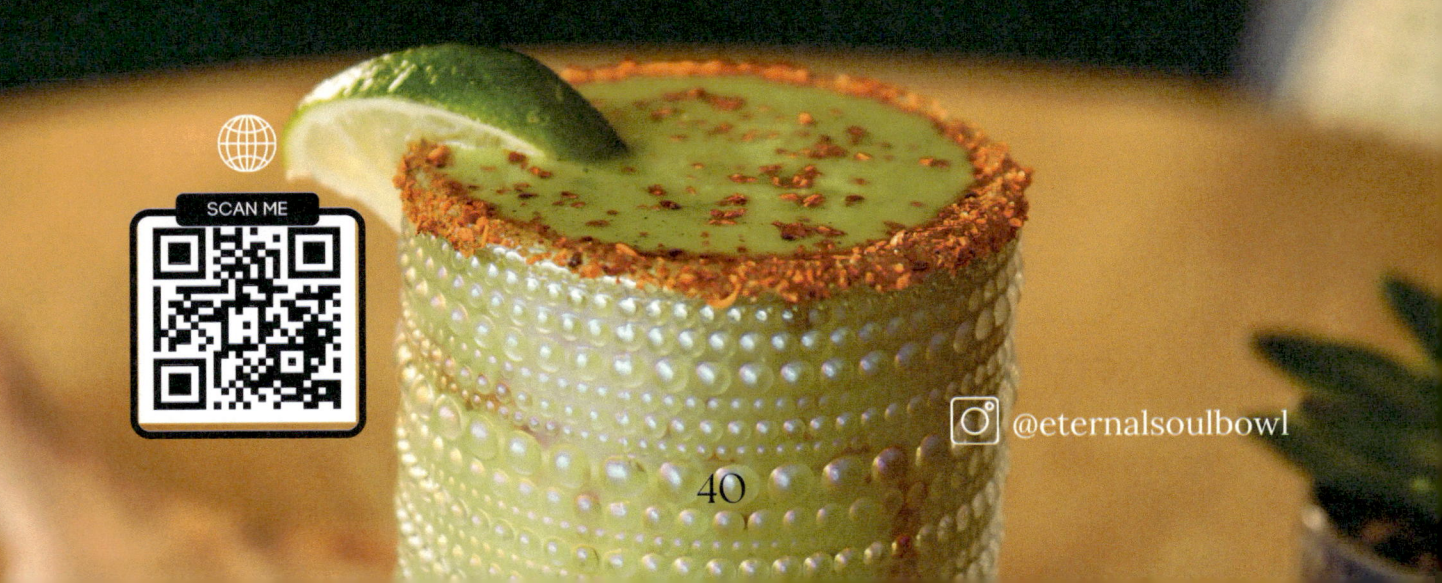

@eternalsoulbowl

41

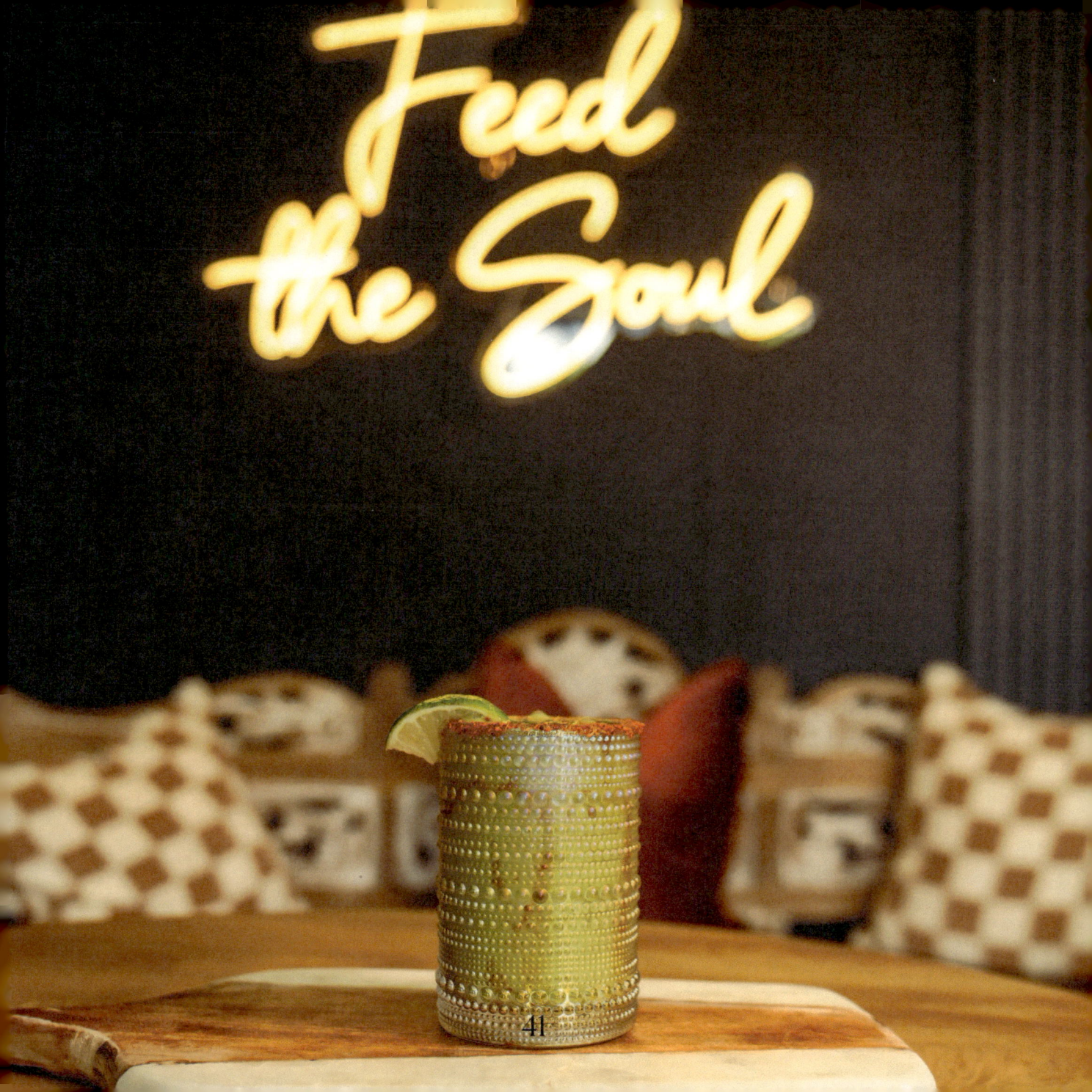

STRAWBERRY MOJITO
Reyna Robyn Photography

Reyna Robyn Photography, located in Bonney Lake, WA, specializes in cocktail and commercial photography. Make sure to explore Reyna's website to discover her collection of other cocktail books available for purchase. Every single image in this book has been skillfully captured by Reyna herself.

Recipe

- 1oz White rum
- 1.5 tbs Fresh lime juice
- 1.5 tbs Simple syrup
- 1 Lime wedge
- 4-5 Fresh mint leaves
- 2 Large strawberries
- Lime Sparkling Water
- 1 cup ice cubes

Barware from: @bleu.grace.home & Pickle Patch at Inta Vintage

Directions

1. Add mint leaves, one large diced strawberry to a glass and muddle
2. Add ice on top of the muddled mint and strawberry.
3. Take a small blender or food processor and add the other large strawberry, rum, lime juice and simple syrup.
4. Blend until smooth. Pour over the ice.
5. Top off with Sparkling water
6. Garnish with Strawberry and fresh mint

www.reynarobynphotography.com

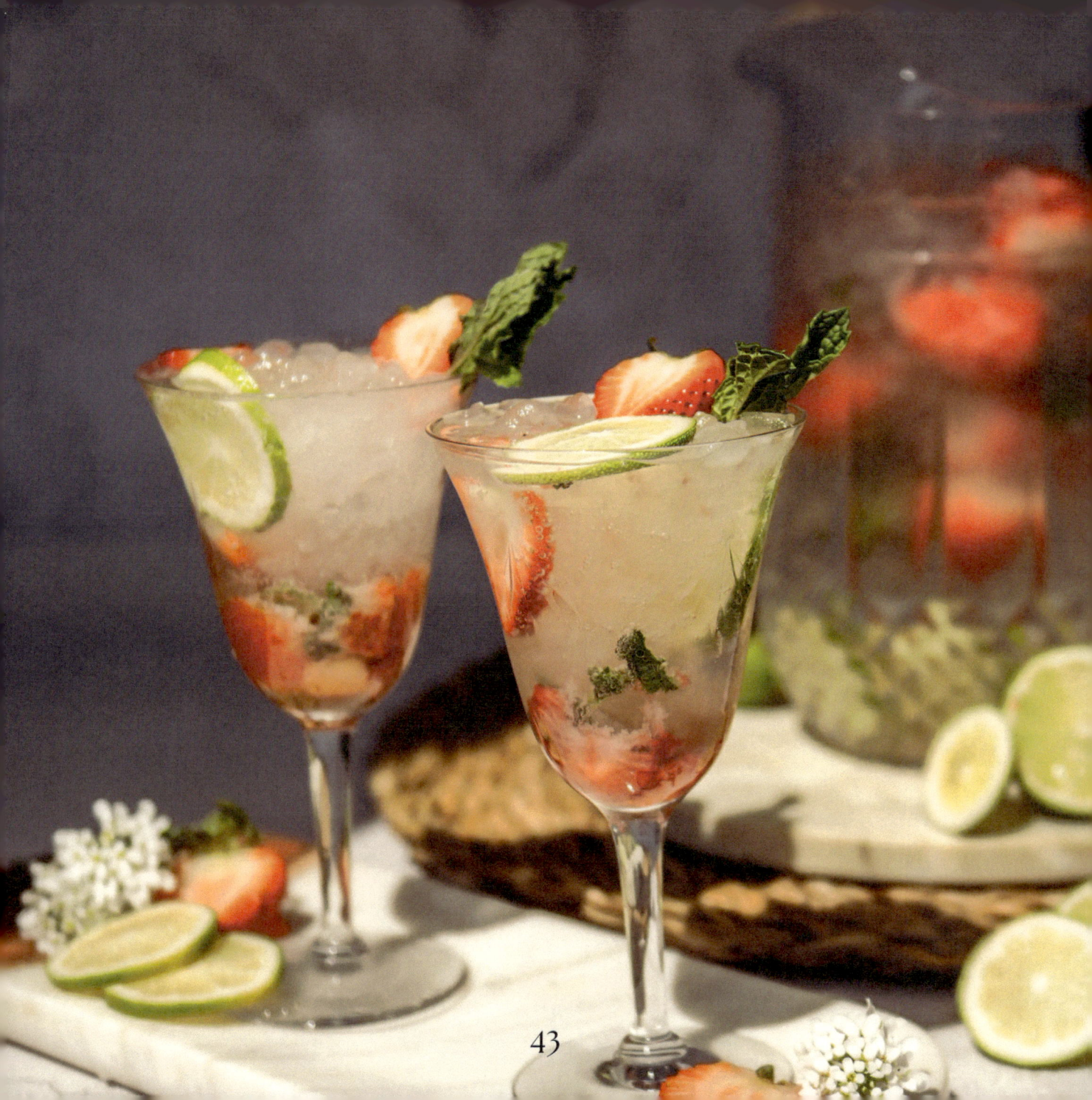

SUMNER MAIN STREET ASSOCIATION

The Sumner Main Street Association is a non-profit organization under Washington Trust for Historic Preservation, whose mission is to create a vibrant and thriving downtown community in Sumner, WA. By partnering with local businesses, community members, and partners- SMSA works to honor history and revitalize our downtown district. Supporting local businesses is at the root of our work, and we are honored to help showcase some of those in our community, while highlighting the farming culture of the Cascade Valley. Rhubarb has a special place in our community and has been grown in our valley for over 100 years. We hope these recipes inspire you to support local farms and raise a glass to tradition. Your support of local businesses, community efforts, and resources is what helps create the special place that is Sumner, WA. Thank you for your love of our small-town and of course... rhubarb.

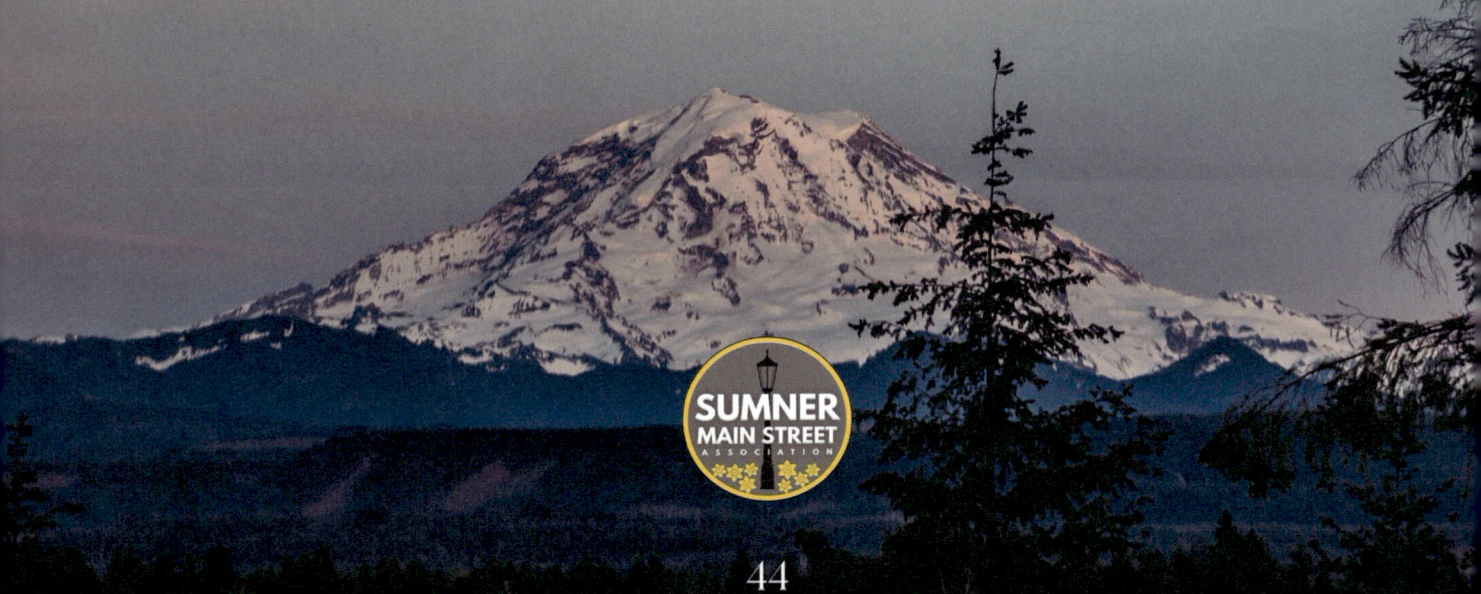

Made in the USA
Columbia, SC
27 July 2024